Building a Five-Star Relationship with Your Horse

The Five Domains of Animal Welfare, when applied to horses, can act as a safe, reliable source of advice and information for conscientious owners, and also a benchmark by which the practices of the more experienced can be measured, scrutinised and held to account. They provide standards to be met rather than levels to be tolerated.

This book explains, in accessible, everyday language, how to apply the Five Domains throughout the horse world, whatever type of equine is concerned or whatever role he or she fulfils, from pet to Thoroughbred racehorse, from informal friend and hack to Olympic competitor. The Domains have been expertly devised, carefully constructed and logically categorised so that anyone can find trustworthy advice on just about any problem or issue they are likely to meet in their lives with horses.

Looking after a horse properly is an excellent way of preventing problems in the first place, and this book provides reliable information on knowing how to assess a horse on a daily and weekly basis so that owners will realise at a glance that something is not quite right or seriously wrong. These skills are accessible and are crucial to responsible, correct horse care and management.

SUSAN McBANE

Building a Five-Star Relationship with Your Horse
Using the Five Domains of Animal Welfare

CRC Press
Taylor & Francis Group
Boca Raton London New York

CRC Press is an imprint of the
Taylor & Francis Group, an **informa** business

Cover credit: Shutterstock

First edition published 2025
by CRC Press
2385 NW Executive Center Drive, Suite 320, Boca Raton FL 33431

and by CRC Press
4 Park Square, Milton Park, Abingdon, Oxon, OX14 4RN

CRC Press is an imprint of Taylor & Francis Group, LLC

ISBN: 978-1-032-49991-8 (hbk)
ISBN: 978-1-032-48874-5 (pbk)
ISBN: 978-1-003-39637-6 (ebk)

DOI: 10.1201/9781003396376

Typeset in Joanna MT
by Apex CoVantage, LLC

Contents

Susan McBane and I have been friends and colleagues for very many years. We have both had considerable experience of horses and have been freelance trainers in the past.

Susan and I, both equestrian authors, started a quarterly, voluntary, non-profit making magazine in 2008. It is a subscription magazine and has never taken advertising, in order that we can remain independent of the commercial world and say what needs to be said on behalf of equines everywhere.

Susan and I share exactly the same ethos of putting the horse's best interests first. Our opinions differ slightly on one or two of the finer points of training, but this is a very healthy situation, and makes us both less likely to hold 'blinkered' opinions.

Susan's writing ability, and love for the horse, is obvious and needs no validation. She has been writing successful horse books for very many years.

This book is a vital addition to any horse lover's library. Its objective is to use The Five Domains of Animal Welfare (formerly known as The Five Freedoms) to give specific equine information as reliable guidance for owners; maybe principally to novice and slightly above, but hopefully for rather more experienced owners as well (who, in my personal view, may well have been 'led astray' by conventional practice and instruction). Following truly horse-friendly ways of managing and riding horses must improve our relationship with them, and that is what the book aims to do.

Anne Wilson

Susan McBane is known worldwide as a long-established equestrian author, this book being her 50th. She has contributed to and revised several other books for publishers and written hundreds of magazine articles. She has an HNC in Equine Science and Management, is a Classical Riding Club listed trainer and Gold Award holder, and an Associate Member of the International Society for Equitation Science.

In 1978, with Dr Moyra Williams, herself an author, clinical psychologist, sport-horse breeder and intrepid horsewoman, Susan founded the Equine Behaviour Study Circle, later re-named the Equine Behaviour Forum, editing its members' journal for 30 years.

Susan has edited two commercial magazines, self-publishing one of them, EQUI, and is currently Publishing Editor of *Tracking-up*, a voluntary, non-profit quarterly which she produces with equestrian teacher and author Anne Wilson (email: annewilsondressage@hotmail.co.uk). Susan taught classical riding for 20 years, for much of that time combining it with Equitation Science, the blending of the two being what she considers to be an ideal system of equitation. She has also acted as an expert witness, consultant, peer reviewer, judge and speaker on equestrian topics.

0.1 A 'ROADMAP' TO SUCCESS

Horse ownership is a dream that, despite our currently poor national economy, more and more people, it seems, are not only aspiring to but achieving. They usually have previous experience of horses and ponies, either at a good riding centre or through family practice, but even so it can be confusing keeping up with modern knowledge and knowing exactly what the most important aspects of horse care and management are to master.

The point of this book is to organise and prioritise the essential knowledge, using a proven system known as The Five Domains of Animal Welfare, and applying them here strictly to horses and ponies. Where do we start, and what knowledge do we need in order to give ourselves the confidence and skills to properly look after and associate with horses, to know when things are going well and when they are not, and whom to consult in the latter instance?

The Five Domains of Animal Welfare clearly set out what we need to know: all we need to do is apply them specifically to horses, which is what this book will be all about. The Five Domains were updated some years ago from the original Five Freedoms of Animal Welfare which were:

Freedom from Hunger and Thirst by ready access to fresh water and a diet to maintain full health and vigour.
Freedom from Discomfort by providing a proper environment, including shelter and a comfortable resting area.
Freedom from Pain, Injury and Disease by provision or rapid diagnosis and treatment.
Freedom to Express Normal Behaviour by providing sufficient space, proper facilities and company of the animal's own kind.
Freedom from Fear and Distress by ensuring conditions and treatment which avoid mental suffering.

DOI: 10.1201/9781003396376-1

The Five Freedoms, a first formal attempt at defining and organising the issue of animal welfare, were excellent as far as they went, but as time went on it was felt that they were perhaps rather passive in their tone and could be improved by being more active and direct, and so the Five Domains of Animal Welfare were devised. There is a great deal of both academic and lay information about them online for anyone interested in their history and application in general. The Five Domains are:

Nutrition: availability and quality of feed and water. (Water intake, food intake and food quality.)

Physical Environment: atmospheric and environmental conditions. (Temperature, confinement, freedom and shelter.)

Health: presence or absence of disease and injury. (Recognition, diagnosis, treatment, prognosis.)

Behavioural Interactions: restriction or expression of behaviour. (Choices and limitations.)

Mental State: subjective feelings and experiences. (Pain/discomfort, thermal comfort, boredom, frustration, fear, happiness.)

There are various 'tweakings' of the Five Domains wherever you look or whatever sources you consult about them, and some experts feel that they are imperfect and lacking in some respects, but the preceding are formal definitions and the main aspects to be considered when associating with and managing animals. The Five Domains will doubtless be updated even more as our Social Licence to Operate (SLO or public acceptance or 'permission') becomes increasingly prominent in the continuance of our relationships with animals, whether in food production, wildlife protection, zoos and parks, companionship or assistance roles, medical and veterinary research and practice, or working and sporting activities.

0.2 HISTORY AND MODERN STATUS

Horses have been a large part of mankind's existence for roughly 6,000 years when it is thought that they were first domesticated in middle and eastern Asia. Initially hunted for food and the numerous useful parts of their bodies such as bone, hide, horn, hair, milk and blood, they gradually became domestically herded and corralled and were eventually harnessed and finally ridden. Over the centuries, mankind has used them for food, transport both ridden and in harness, war, entertainment, mounted hunting, sport and industry. Horses, mules and asses/donkeys are still an economic necessity in many developing countries of the world and work for their living elsewhere in Europe, Asia, America, Australasia and Africa, experiencing very varied welfare standards. (Further details of this aspect are available from the charity World Horse Welfare.)

Modern attitudes to animals are geared much more towards welfare and well-being than formerly. This book is specifically about horses and ponies, one of whose main connections with humans today being sport, mostly competitive sport. Millions of people, however, keep equines to ride and associate with non-competitively as friends, companions and rather large pets and retirees. Breeding racehorses and competition horses has been a lucrative and economically important endeavour for generations, the competition element having burgeoned after the Second World War and, in westernised countries, athletic competitions and showing, at all levels, are probably horses' main roles.

0.3 THE FUTURE

It has been suggested that, if the horse world does not improve its implementation of welfare criteria and standards of equine well-being in all areas of the horse world in the near future, in 20 years' time we shall no longer be legally allowed to ride or drive equines. There is also the issue of equines being used as pack and harness animals in some developing countries – there is no reason to suppose that the current SLO will only be recognised in the United Kingdom.

Of course, being prevented from riding horses is unthinkable to many horse people, but we have already seen public opinion effectively bring about the legal banning of animals on circuses in Britain and the cessation of mounted hunting of foxes, hares and deer, trail or drag hunting still being permitted.

The very act of confining, handling, training and working horses can cause them distress in many ways, from universally too-early weaning; inappropriate handling; living in isolation; incomprehensible vocal commands; inconsistent and therefore confusing 'aids', cues and signals aimed at instructing and controlling horses; painful application of whips, spurs and bits; uncomfortable and even painful accoutrements such as saddles, bridles, headgear, clothing and leg wear; unwanted (by the horse) attentions from vets and farriers; confinement; artificial breeding; separation from friends; enforced proximity to unfriendly horses; transportation; inhumane euthanasia; inappropriate management practices – the list goes on.

Some people truly do not realise that they are being unfair or even cruel to their horses, due to lack of education in their mentality, physiology, care and management. Economic conditions, in Britain and other countries, have seen the closure of many excellent riding schools where previous generations could go to gain essential experience and knowledge. Yet owning a horse has not decreased in popularity: indeed, many who would have ridden at a local riding school now have their own horses instead, often kept at sub-standard livery yards on a DIY basis and using largely social media for often-dubious advice and information regarding all aspects of how to deal with them and care for them. Conventional riding lessons also often promote methods proven by modern Equitation Science to be inappropriate to horses' mentalities, physiques and care requirements.

Livery yard proprietors are, also, often from a farming background, diversifying into equine livery for economic reasons, and may not have the requisite species knowledge to advise their customers about their horses. Some yard owners often provide inadequate facilities for horses, usually on a take-it-or-leave-it basis. Many yards are no more than DIY rental yards, without even a competent manager to look out for the horses' welfare.

Unfortunately, it cannot be denied that there are many experienced horse people who do not have an appropriate attitude to their involvement with horses where the horses' welfare is concerned. Many well-known equestrians are keen to be seen and heard using such familiar phrases as 'the horses' welfare is paramount' when, to the knowledgeable observer, it plainly is not. I hope that the plain, basic information in this book will help all horse enthusiasts to be able to tell when and whether horses and ponies are being well looked after, no matter what those in charge of them say.

Very many horses kept for the convenience of their human connections in unsuitable environments and under inappropriate management and work conditions suffer from stereotypical behaviours, formerly known as 'stable vices', self-inflicted injuries and psychological, behavioural problems which can be incurable. A slaughterhouse owner told me as far back as the early 1990s that more horses were put down by him at that time from behavioural issues than ever before because owners were 'pale shadows' of their knowledgeable and genuinely compassionate predecessors who were brought up in an equine environment and understood and cared about their horses.

0.4 WHAT TO DO?

The Five Domains of Animal Welfare, when applied to horses, can act as both a safe, reliable source of advice and information for conscientious owners, and also a benchmark by which the practices of the more experienced can be measured, scrutinised and held to account. They provide standards to be met rather than levels to be tolerated.

They will work throughout the horse world, whatever type of horse or pony is concerned or whatever role he or she fulfils, from pet to Thoroughbred racehorse, competitive showjumper or eventer or driving horse to informal friend and hack, or from Olympic competitor to child's pony or retired family member, or to working equines in some developing countries. The Domains have been expertly devised, carefully constructed and logically categorised so that anyone, whatever type of equine they have, can understand them and use them as a framework for effective and appropriate dealings with their horses and ponies. They help them to find trustworthy advice on just about any problem or issue they are likely to meet in their lives with horses. Recognising a problem is half-way to solving it, and knowing what kind of expert or practitioner can solve it is essential to the future well-being of both horse and owner. Information on this is given in the book.

Looking after, handling and working a horse properly, though, is an excellent way of preventing problems in the first place and this book gives reliable information on knowing how to assess a horse, knowing and developing 'feel' for horses, so that owners will realise when something is not quite right or is seriously wrong, and knowing whom to trust to consult on their horse's well-being. These skills are accessible and are crucial to responsible, correct horse care and management.

As mentioned earlier, social media is, often unfortunately, many owners' first port of call when they have a query about their horse or pony. This can work quite well, if also being rather confusing should they consult more than one 'advisor'. However, I firmly believe that, so far as an animal's well-being is concerned, it is very well worthwhile to pay to consult a vet. Or other appropriate expert. I know this can add to one's expenses, but welfare is at the root of everything and really must not be skimped.

The three main experts needed to help owners and carers to understand and look after horses and ponies in their charge are an equine veterinary surgeon, an equine nutritionist and a farrier. Others include an equine dentist/dental technician, a physiotherapist, a massage therapist, a saddle and bridle fitter and, increasingly, an equine behavioural therapist. All these experts should be qualified by recognised organisations.

Another requirement is to buy yourself up-to-date text books on various aspects of horse care and management, specifically veterinary matters, equine nutrition, farriery, tack and behaviour/psychology. Whether or not you want to take examinations in these topics, they will act as an excellent basis for your own knowledge and ongoing experience and, crucially, will help you to know when to consult a relevant, true expert. At the end of the day, when in doubt do the latter.

0.5 THE STRUCTURE OF THIS BOOK

The book is arranged in sections rather than chapters – one for each Domain. The main topics covered in each section are as follows.

First Domain – Nutrition: digestive system from teeth to faeces and urine; natural and 'artificial' foods; poisonous plants and other 'eatables'; types and quality of foodstuffs; amounts and types needed for health and occupation; a 'balanced diet'; mechanics of food and water provision for eating and drinking comfort; recognising feeding-related disorders such as colic, laminitis, allergies, choke, excess or insufficient energy, dental issues, bodyweight and condition.

Second Domain – Physical environment: equine society and relationships; the Equitation Science 'Three F's – Friends, Freedom and Foraging'; the outdoor life, pros, cons and facilities; indoor accommodation from individual stabling to group housing, good and bad; air quality and provision; a safe environment; volume and type of noise; confinement; freedom; shelter; ground conditions and footing, indoors and out; rugs, tack and other equipment.

Third Domain – Health: recognising good health and condition (bodyweight); recognising illness, injury, lameness and mental disorders such as stereotypical behaviour; daily and weekly checks and records; first aid versus veterinary interventions; when to call the vet; handling sick, frightened and injured horses; diagnosis methods; prognosis; retirement for better or worse; euthanasia.

Fourth Domain – Behavioural interactions: restriction, two sides of the coin; equine behavioural expression; is it our fault and can we help?; interactions with humans, horses and other species; giving the horse choices in life; learned helplessness; limitations on behavioural expression; how to ameliorate poor conditions.

Fifth Domain – Mental state: causes of subjective feelings; the effects of experiences; causes of pain and discomfort and how to help alleviate them; equine emotional expression; calmness – horses' natural state;

boredom; frustration; happiness; sadness; anxiety; fear; anticipation; confidence; horses' temperature tolerances.

In addition: topics which do not fit easily into any of the Five Domains are also discussed briefly, such as general treatment of and expectations from horses, travelling, training, working, competing, breeding, buying and selling, the 'user' mentality and the horse as a commodity.

The Five Domains are, to older generations, a relatively new development in horse care and riding and, while no one can deny the impact on the horse world of increasing public pressure to improve equine welfare and general well-being, that alone is insufficient reason to try to keep up to date with not only modern opinions but also today's vastly increased and improved knowledge in all aspects of looking after and working with horses. Well-cared for and trained horses enrich the lives of not only those who associate with them but also those who simply love watching them in their various jobs, or even just loafing around with each other in a field.

Horses have a unique place in our societies. Their status is on a par with that of dogs, cats and other animals commonly held to be pets and companions, yet they often work hard for us; earn money for us; are very expensive to breed, buy and maintain properly; and have that unusual combination of qualities of being both 'work-horses' and close friends at the same time. In some countries, horses are bred for food both human and animal: that is no excuse to treat them inhumanely during their lifetimes, the same going for any farmed creature, of course.

The Five Domains applied to horses offer a clear guide and reference that, correctly used, will safeguard equestrianism, expose those who fall short in their care and use of horses, and ensure the practical well-being and welfare of our horses and ponies.

Nutrition

One

The saying 'eats like a horse' gives even non-horsey people a good idea of the amount of food horses eat. The equine digestive system is in use for nearly all of the horse's 24 hours. We human omnivores (meaning we can eat all types of food) are currently being bombarded in magazines and television programmes with the topic of fasting – how good it can be for us, particularly those of us who eat a good deal of meat and red meat at that. Not so horses and other herbivores who eat only vegetation of various sorts.

The horse's digestive system evolved to have food passing through it for most of the time because vegetation is less nutrient-rich than flesh, even in spring. If a horse's digestive system goes without any food at all for very close to four continuous hours, it becomes compromised, as acidic digestive juices are still secreted which can cause damage to the sensitive stomach and intestines, cause the horse to feel unwell and encourage him to experiment with whatever is within reach. Some people complain that their horse's behaviour is 'ratty', that he eats his bedding (even shavings if he is that desperate), chews wood when he can reach it and snatches at food very determinedly when being ridden: these are all signs of unnatural hunger due to a horse-unfriendly diet. There may be times when he has to be kept without food, such as before an operation at the vet's, but generally speaking, horses need to be able to 'trickle feed' almost continuously in order to take in and process the amount of nourishment they need over 24 hours.

We may be familiar with horses being 'starved' before work by old-fashioned or less knowledgeable people, leaving them without food sometimes for two hours or more because they genuinely believe that working them on a 'full stomach' will cause indigestion and colic. This old idea still persists in environments where horse-keepers have not kept up to date. Doubtless things will change as research continues but, generally, food may be removed an hour or two before hard and/or fast work, but half an hour *before* that work starts horses – and this goes for

DOI: 10.1201/9781003396376-2

working ponies, too – a small roughage feed should be given of chop (chopped-up hay with perhaps a little straw) to help 'soak up' digestive juices that may be splashed around by activity and damage the delicate stomach lining. It will also help the horse to feel better than being hungry. (The word 'chop' is the correct description for this type of feed. The word 'chaff' is often used but, strictly, chaff is part of the inside husk of grain, not chopped hay.)

1.1 DIGESTION

We probably all know how mobile and strong a horse's lips are. They are vital to enable the horse to sort out available food and gather it into his mouth. The front teeth or incisors also grab food for the muscular tongue and back teeth to deal with. The tongue moves the food around as saliva is produced to soften it up and the mighty, rough back teeth (the pre-molars and molars) crush and grind it up to make it easy for the horse to swallow.

The food, obviously, passes down from the mouth where saliva starts the 'softening up' process, down the 'food pipe' or oesophagus and into the stomach where strong, acidic digestive juices, buffered by the alkaline saliva, break it down further. The circular sphincter muscle at the entrance to the stomach prevents the horse being sick, which must be regarded as a disadvantage because if the horse or pony eats anything that disagrees with it serious illness can result. Colic is not dreaded for nothing.

The food passes along the voluminous, compartmentalised tube into the belly where most of the digestion process takes place. The horse, like us, needs vitamins, minerals, protein, carbohydrate and fats and other substances, and the pancreas and liver are crucially involved with the process of digestion. The unused, waste 'food' is pushed out of the anus under the horse's tail as the droppings we are all so familiar with.

Water is also obviously essential, and horses will need from five to ten gallons of water per day or roughly 23 to 46 litres or more but, like humans and other mammals, much depends on the weather, temperature, exercise or work, and it is important that the horse has ready access to as much water as he needs over his day and night. Water is essential to maintain the body's fluid balance to enable it to function properly and produce hormones and other essential substances, and it needs to be clean, fresh and readily available (in a regularly cleaned-out container) otherwise the horse may well not drink enough to maintain his health not to mention his comfort.

Droppings and urine can tell us a good bit about a horse's general health. If a horse is fed on mainly hay, grain and/or pelleted food the droppings will be moist balls which just break on hitting the ground. Their colour will be brownish. A horse or pony eating more grass will produce greenish droppings, softer than those of a stabled horse. If droppings are small and/or hard, this indicates constipation and if they are very soft or not formed at all, of course it indicates diarrhoea. If there is blood in the droppings or they are any colour other than brownish to greenish, there could be a significant problem requiring a call to the vet. Urine is yellowish in colour, pale and clear or slightly cloudy, again with no blood in it. Both have a distinctive but not an offensive smell in the healthy horse. If a horse has difficulty passing faeces or urine, or either smells acrid or otherwise strong or unpleasant, this would certainly need a call to the vet.

1.2 NATURAL OR 'MAN-MADE'?

Here is a little story I have told before but which stands telling again. Decades ago, I used to write for a professional magazine produced for riding schools and commercial equestrian businesses. They also had writing for them a gentleman who was a well-respected and vastly experienced horseman. This tale comes from him.

During the Second World War, many leisure activities were curtailed in Britain and food, of course, was rationed for both humans and animals. Horses were not allowed oats – the traditional 'work' food for equines – because they were reserved for humans. Without 'hard' food, people worried about how their horses would be kept fit for work and play, hunting still going on: they had little choice but to feed them the very best quality hay they could find, along with whatever root vegetables they could acquire and that the horses would eat, and grass according to circumstances.

Hunters generally were allowed to eat as much top quality hay as they wanted and, even without their oats, managed very well to still do their four days a fortnight hunting in winter with no noticeable deterioration in performance or condition.

This was, of course, long before 'horse nuts' (cubes or bagged, commercial feeds) had been invented. Nowadays, we are so used to commercial and professionally produced specialist horse feeds that we panic if we cannot find our favourite brand. (All changes to diet need to be made gradually, of course, over two to four weeks or so, to allow the horse's system to register the change and produce appropriate digestive juices for a different feed. Many people also do not realise that the relatively large number of overweight horses and ponies, not to mention the vastly increased number of laminitis cases compared with decades ago, were simply not seen by previous generations of horse and pony owners. None of this is the fault of the feed manufacturers, of course, but the tendency of many owners to over-feed their animals on concentrated, manufactured feeds and regard them as the most important part of their diet.

May I, yet again, stick my neck out and say that all my decades of experience with everything from small ponies to Thoroughbred racehorses and heavy horses has convinced and confirmed to me that, with rare exceptions, concentrate feeds, whether oats, barley, cubes or whatever else, are not the most crucial part of a horse's diet. That honour goes to hay and haylage. Of course, they need to be of the right sort and nutrient content for the animal in question. Haylage has become increasingly popular for horses in recent decades, and most horses do love it: this could be partly because it is, of course, a moist feed whereas hay, unless wet or soaked, is dry and less comfortable to eat. Quite a few horses dunk their hay in their water container to overcome this situation, and they should not be prevented from doing this. If it annoys their carers, the hay should be soaked or wetted before feeding.

Grazing grass and browsing shrubbery and trees for their leaves is obviously the horse's natural occupation for most of every day and well-made hay and/or haylage is the first step in the formulation of an 'artificial' diet for them. Top class forage like this of the right type for the horse or pony concerned is a gift from Heaven. They eat it well and willingly and thrive wonderfully on it. I believe it must form the basis of the ideal diet for horses not on grass much the time.

That is not to say, of course, that concentrate feeds of various kinds are not needed, depending on the horse or pony's type and workload, but start with the best appropriate hay/haylage you can get. Build up from there with grains such as rolled oats or bruised barley here in the UK or whatever natural concentrate feeds are used in your country, or commercial, bagged feeds. Most good feed companies give customers free access to expert advice via a freephone number (and not only on their products), so it is not difficult or expensive to devise the ideal diet for your horse or pony, with ongoing support from an expert professional.

Feeds containing grain are best mixed with chop (good quality hay or haylage chopped short), maybe with some straw (preferably oat) added, and also bran, which is part of the inner husk of wheat grains. These traditional additions make a feed bulkier and larger, add variety and aid digestion. Many people also add a little salt also to a feed. All these practices can be discussed with your nutritionist. Grated roots such as carrots are also very welcome, but hard roots must not be fed in chunks because of the risk of choking.

Although commercial feed companies do not normally sell hay or haylage, these being sold mainly by their makers, their specialist equine nutritionists can advise you on the feed content and the type of forage you should be looking for for your horse or pony. Many growers now have their products professionally analysed before selling them so that they can give this information to customers and to any nutritionist advising them, so they are able to supply different feed grades of forage, so do ask about this when looking for a supply of forage, a term which covers both hay and haylage.

As for grass itself, what equine does not love getting its head down among the green stuff. It is what he evolved for and it is Horse Heaven – but we all know that not all types of grass suit all types of equine. Laminitis is excruciatingly painful, foot-deforming and life-threatening. It can come on very quickly and, once bitten, an animal can get it again and again. Although most of us know that long grass, particularly sugar-rich ryegrass or milk-cow pasture, is dangerous to horses in this respect, very short-grazed land is not the answer. Over-grazed land produces stressed grass which, itself, can bring on laminitis due to the high levels of non-structural carbohydrates it contains. The horse or pony's body releases insulin in response, and laminitis is the result.

Livery clients may have little or no choice in what grass is available to their horse, but if it is long and lush ration your animal's time on it. Sugar rises in grass during daylight hours so it is best, if at all possible, to have susceptible horses and ponies turned out during the night and brought in as soon as possible in the morning, being turned out again at night. An alternative regime would be to have them turned out early in the morning and brought in at mid-morning, with additional time out during the evening.

Laminitis is the subject of ongoing research because it is still not fully understood. Bear in mind, though, that it is a killer and extremely painful, so we should do everything we can to avoid triggering it.

Poisonous plants from grass to trees and all points in between can also be fatal. Depending on your country, it's good to search the internet or buy a veterinary or specialist book on what grows in your country that could kill your horse: you might get some surprises. Any symptoms such as colic-like signs, staggering, groaning, frequent rolling, collapsing, lying down a good deal, salivating or, indeed, anything abnormal could indicate poisoning and need rapid veterinary attention.

1.3 HOW MUCH OF WHAT?

In what we call the 'developed world', the main mistake regarding feeding horses and especially ponies is over-feeding whereas in other countries charities constantly deal with working animals that are under-nourished, weak and even starving. A quick, reliable guide to healthy bodyweight is that you should be able to easily feel an animal's ribs but not see them, unless he is turning away from you. Any sign of a big, 'pot' belly with a poor covering of flesh over the top of the horse (from poll to tail) also indicates very poor nutrition.

Because horses naturally need to have food passing through them most of the time, the objective is generally to feed as much good quality, appropriate hay as the horse wants, with concentrates added if extra energy or nutrition is needed. 'Good quality' does not necessarily mean a high nutrient content but that the hay is clean (not dusty or mouldy) and smells sweet and appetising. Meadow hay with many different types of grasses in it is excellent for most horses and ponies, and they usually love it. Higher nutrient hay, mostly higher-sugar/carbohydrate ryegrass hay, is often used for hard-working horses.

It's true that some horses, like many people, eat more food than they need for health and work, so use the bodyweight guide above to keep an eye on your horse's intake. Checking your horse or pony's condition weekly with a weigh-tape is a reliable, standard way of keeping a close eye on his condition. Fasting is not the way to control bodyweight in horses except on veterinary advice. I think it is true to say that many horses are perilously short of food overnight, particularly on livery yards that ban owners from early or mid-evening and do not feed their horses for them later at night. This causes not only mental discontent but also considerable physical discomfort and is outright bad horse management to the point of cruelty. If necessary because of such conditions, it is better to feed more of a good, clean but lower nutrient-content hay so that the horse does not go over the maximum of four hours without food.

To bulk out hay, for this reason or at times of shortage, clean oat straw can be added to the hay container and mixed with the hay. This will add bulk without excess nutrients and is something to discuss with a nutritionist or vet as to appropriate proportions for your horse or pony. Straw can cause intestinal blockages in small ponies.

Roots are nearly always welcomed by horses, especially carrots and apples although not all like things like beets or turnips. Adding something juicy like this to most or each feed will be welcomed by the horse and large roots can be given between feeds as a nutritious treat that will also give a horse some occupation. Slightly damping feeds just before feeding is a good practice. If feeds are damped too soon they can turn sour tasting and may well not be eaten. Should you soak or damp hay or not? If it is of good quality this should not be necessary, although many horses seem to prefer damp or wet hay, as mentioned earlier.

1.4 JUDGING QUALITY

Feed of any kind may well have a distinctive smell of its own, but no feed should smell musty or sour. There should be no sign of mould, dust or any foreign material present.

Good hay of any kind has a wonderful, sweet aroma, is clean and easy to separate for feeding. Hay that is clumped together, that smells anything other than sweet or is obviously dusty or mouldy should never be fed. It would be better to pay out for bagged, chopped forage (hay, straw and other items chosen by the manufacturer) than to risk your horse's health – if he will eat rubbish at all and some will! When you shake out hay before feeding, there should not be any dust coming from it. Haylage similarly should smell sweet and inviting, not sour in any way.

Concentrate feeds, whether natural grains such as slightly crushed (rolled) oats or barley or commercially made, branded and bagged feed, loose or as 'nuts', should also be clean, dry, easily separated and with no suspicious smell or sign of dampness.

1.5 STORAGE

Where you keep your horse's feed can affect its quality long-term. All feed, whether loose or bagged, can be badly affected to the point of being ruined by exposure to wet or damp which will cause it to deteriorate quickly. Rats and mice, of course, looking for a home in your hay, for instance, can taint it with their body smell, and their urine and faeces, so measures to keep them away should be in place. Tidy habits to discourage them, such as keeping feed bins properly closed and clearing up any spills, should be followed.

Hay in particular needs to be in an airy, dry storage area: open-fronted barns with their entrances facing away from the prevailing wind are good with the hay kept as far to the back of the barn as possible, ideally with air circulating around it, to avoid wetting from rain or snow. Haylage normally comes bagged and is easier to store.

Other feeds are usually bought in jute sacks or, if from a specialist feed firm, plastic or, increasingly, paper sacks. Obviously, these, too, must be kept in dry conditions. Plastic or metal bins, with lids, are common although rats can chew through some plastic bins. After one load of feed is used up, the bin should be cleaned out with plain water and dried before refilling.

1.6 SUPPLEMENTS

Nutrient supplements, usually vitamins and minerals, can be useful in certain cases on the advice of a nutritionist or vet, such as building up a sick or thin horse or one in hard work, but mainly they seem to be used too often, and unnecessarily if a good, basic diet is being fed. The subject of nutritional balance is very complicated, and it is not feasible, for most people, to get every sample of new feed analysed. Hay, a stock of which may last months, can usefully be analysed, commercial feeds will have their analysis on the sack, and good samples of natural barley, maize or oat grains will have standard contents which you can discuss with a nutritionist.

(If you buy your hay fresh-cut off the field, remember it will take a few months to mature or 'make' to be ready to feed and needs to be stored in well-ventilated conditions meanwhile.)

Adding a supplement to good quality feed can actually unbalance it. Having said that, horses in hard, specialist work such as racing or endurance may well gain an extra nutritional 'edge' by means of a good supplement, but it is a good plan to discuss this with a nutritionist or vet before going ahead. The idea is to give your horse what he needs for his work and health: overdoing it may actually cause ill health.

1.7 DELIVERING THE GOODS

By nature, horses like to search out (forage for) their own food. Of course, they crop grass and leaves with their front teeth as described earlier, taken from natural conditions. Delivering feed and water to horses can be an art in itself. Some horses will not eat or drink out of certain containers. I used to have a horse who ripped every haynet he was given when the hay ran out so we had to, rather wastefully, feed it in a corner on the ground as the yard owner would not permit us to install any kind of rack.

Feed containers for stables vary considerably. Not every horse can be trusted to not knock over a bucket of feed (or, indeed, water), losing most of it in his bedding. I have always liked triangular mangers fixed in a corner, although I knew a horse who would always lift his manger out of its frame and put it on the floor without upsetting it. Any manger has to be carefully sited so that the horse can eat with his poll lower than his withers as nature dictates but without the chance of bruising his knees on the lower edge of the manger. Some horses continually stamp when eating or stand on one foreleg, waving the other around. Some scoop out the feed with their muzzles and waste it unless your box is big enough to sacrifice a feeding corner with no bedding in it, where the horse can easily clean up. They all have their mannerisms: if you are lucky you may have a horse who will eat peacefully from a bucket on the ground and not waste a single grain or nut.

It is amazing how sensitive and manipulative horses' lips are, but we should not be surprised at this because they are their life-support system. Many horses are quite capable of wheedling out their favourite items in a bucket of mixed ingredients as small as grains, leaving the less favoured ones in the manger. Sorting out their favourite grasses from pasture or hay is also easy for them. The addition of medicine of some kind, a new type of feed or anything unfamiliar can mean the horse will not eat it, which is not good for his health or his owner's bank balance. This is but one reason any changes should be made gradually over days or weeks depending on the amounts of the new addition. The other important reason is that the horse's digestive system needs time to adjust to the new digestive requirements and produce the right elements to cope with it along his digestive tract.

A horse's natural way of eating is mainly with his poll below his withers and his head extended in line with his lowered neck, so the food is swallowed easily up a fairly straight tube (the oesophagus) and passes down into the stomach. A major fault, I find, in any stable yard today is feed containers and buckets or mangers that are too high to allow the horses a comfortable eating and drinking position of the head and neck. This can result in horses not eating enough, not enjoying the process of eating (which in nature they do for well over half their 24 hours), so not being relaxed but discontented most of the time, which is obviously not at all good for their health. Food may not be chewed properly, so possibly causing digestive problems, even colic.

Hay containers, therefore, should be around head height or, preferably, in a large, fixed tub or basket-type container on the ground. If they are too high bits of hay and seeds can fall into the horses' eyes, as well as creating an uncomfortable eating position. It is worth considering, too, the uneven development of the horse's neck muscles as he constantly pulls out the hay. Short-feed containers, whether buckets or fixed mangers, should allow the horse to eat with his poll below his withers, as mentioned. Although horses in nature both graze (from ground level) and browse leaves from trees and shrubs (above average head height), their long necks and heads allow this and their eating positions are very varied. They will pull down leaves and twigs and then lower their heads to eat them comfortably. The action of grazing from the ground (which they enjoy for most of their day, when allowed) is a mentally therapeutic occupation for horses and, generally, should be encouraged rather than prevented.

A structure of a feed container that is strong and solid and goes right to floor level is a good container for 'active' horses, but whatever type of holder you choose, according to your horse's habits, it must be inviting (roomy enough) and safe. A good arrangement is to have firmly fixed or built-in mangers that can be quickly cleaned out with a sponge after feeding. If you use any 'product' to clean any manger, it must be really well rinsed afterwards to remove any unpleasant taste or smell.

Piling the hay loose in a corner is the only safe way of giving it for some horses, although some will probably end up mixed with the bedding.

The point is, we must cater to what our horse wants: he must be comfortable eating and drinking or his digestion could be adversely affected, even if he does not actually colic. Our horses, however much we love them, are prisoners. They tell us as best they can what they want and need. Eating and drinking are of prime importance to them and, if they are correctly managed, they will spend most of their time eating, so surely we must make certain they are as comfortable as possible while doing so. Both feed and water containers need to be sited so that the horse eats and drinks naturally, with his poll lower than his withers, as stressed earlier. This is particularly important for water, otherwise the horse may leave himself short of water because of the discomfort of swallowing with his head too high.

1.8 BEFORE WORK ...

As mentioned earlier, it is, of course, good practice to deprive horses of food before work, even a gentle hack. How long this break should be varies, I find. Half an hour is common, or an hour, but the present advice seems to be no longer than that. A small amount of food can be given then, according to the nature of the work. Remember that horses out at grass, feral or domesticated, will be walking around all the time with their bellies full, and will break into faster gaits now and then either playing or avoiding trouble. If equids are chased by a predator or marauding dog, wolf or lion, they will be galloping fast to evade it and few, if any, of them will go down with colic. The species would soon become extinct otherwise.

1.9 ... AND AFTER

It is best to allow a horse to calm and cool down after his work before feeding. Good practice is to walk him around or walk him home for a good 20 minutes to cool down and before feeding. This is a good chance to let him graze in hand as he will surely be peckish after his work stint. Some people will not allow water for an hour or so, either, but this old practice is not good management. The horse should be allowed repeated, short drinks of about three or four swallows while cooling down, which you will notice if you watch racing on television. I have then always let a horse drink whenever he wants within reason and without any problem after he has cooled down and never had any trouble. Small drinks of a few swallows, including out hacking, are welcome if the horse wants them and have never caused harm in my experience. Some horses will not eat happily or comfortably if they cannot not drink as well after every few mouthfuls of feed, and again, I have never found horses like this to have any ill effects.

1.10 A 'BALANCED' DIET

It is impossible for an 'ordinary' horse or pony owner to be able to understand whether the food their equine is receiving is balanced when it comes to vitamins and minerals. This is where good, commercial feeds come in. Their analyses will be printed on the sack and, although you may still not fully understand their significance, they provide a standard for that type of feed to comply with. I have already recommended that owners take full advantage of the free service available from good feed manufacturers, by freephone, and given by a qualified nutritionist.

Some people do still feed the 'old', traditional way of mixing separate ingredients at home, such as grains like oats, barley or cooked, flaked maize and adding chop (see earlier) and bran. It was less likely, when this method of feeding was common, that horses were, indeed, receiving a balanced diet because people were not so aware of its importance, or of the bad effects possible from too much or too little of particular vitamins or minerals. Having said that, they were still made fit, well and, I am certain, had longer working lives decades ago.

That said, feeding a scientifically formulated feed of varied, high quality ingredients can only be good for your animal provided you choose one meant for his type and work, and feed appropriate quantities regularly in a way he finds easy to cope with. If you can take things a step further and obtain the analysis of your horse's hay or haylage, this will also help the nutritionist to recommend the most suitable feed, and amounts, for your animal. With access to nutritionists, and the quality of commercial feeds, plus a source of really good hay or haylage appropriate for your horses and ponies, there is no need to worry about whether or not they are receiving a balanced diet.

1.11 RECOGNISING FEEDING-RELATED DISORDERS

One of the most serious, painful and, indeed, life-threatening conditions related to feeding is the dreaded colic. Colic is a very serious form of indigestion. The only way you can suspect colic is through your horse's behaviour and this is one excellent reason to get used to your horse's normal demeanour.

The signs of colic in horses or ponies are: a general air of unease, usually standing with the head and neck stretched out a little and maybe held downwards, often with the ears back, turning and snatching at their sides, pawing the ground or bedding, moaning and groaning, maybe leaning on the walls of the stable, rolling often and perhaps 'strongly' or just repeatedly getting down and up again. *It is absolutely essential that, even if these signs are intermittent, you get a vet to come out and see your horse or pony if you suspect colic as it is extremely painful and can often be fatal.*

Laminitis ('fever in the feet') is another very painful and life-threatening condition, and it can come on very quickly indeed. The forefeet are most commonly affected, but any foot or all feet can be affected. Feeding-related triggers of laminitis include too much concentrated feed or sudden changes in diet which do not allow the digestive elements of the digestive system to adapt, sudden increase of starches/carbohydrates in the feed, too much sugar from grain/concentrates or rich grazing. If making any changes in the diet, introduce the new feed very gradually, even a handful only at first, in the existing ration, and increase over, say, a week to a month depending on the amount to be fed.

Signs of laminitis include: uneasiness on the feet with the horse or pony changing weight-bearing on the feet constantly, standing back on the heels, particularly on to the back feet to take the weight off the front ones although laminitis can occur in front and hind feet, reluctance or refusal to walk at all, or even to stand up, an uneasy expression on the face sometimes with groaning and quicker or deeper breathing – a general sign of pain. *Again, urgent veterinary attention is essential.*

Allergies sometimes occur, usually in relation to feed. They can produce various signs, but itchy skin and difficulty in breathing are common. Mostly we are warned to make changes in feeding gradually, but, in the case of allergies, a vet should be consulted and the advice may well be to stop the feed immediately and put the horse on a bland diet with small amounts of familiar concentrates or none at all.

It is the fashion at present to use all sorts of 'products' on horses in the form of shampoos, coat conditioners and so on, rather than letting good health and thorough grooming shine through. If the horse's skin becomes itchy, blotchy or has swollen areas or it breaks out into sores, and certainly if the horse is biting at himself excessively, obviously stop using the product and consult your vet as to, say, anti-inflammatory treatment and possibly an anti-inflammatory shampoo. I think horses are washed too much these days and not groomed properly instead, but if you do want to wash your sensitive horse just use a shampoo or wash designed for human babies and rinse thoroughly, especially under his chest and belly and between the hind legs, where the skin is thinnest.

Choke is one of the most frightening things to happen to a horse, both for the horse and those witnessing it. In horses, choke does not usually interfere with breathing as it does in humans, but it is still a potentially dangerous, emergency situation. Although massaging the throat is sometimes recommended, squirting water into the mouth and other actions are often advised by non-vets, and these are likely to make matters worse.

Ring your vet at once. Even if the horse has cleared the blockage himself quickly, your vet will not be annoyed at your call. Try to keep the horse's head down as this will put the oesophagus (food channel) in a better position for the lump of food to possibly be swallowed. Remove all other food and water and do not replace it until the vet says it is safe to do so. Try to keep the horse calm and with his head down and wait for the vet: obviously, if he or she gives you any instructions over the phone, follow them.

Causes of choke include dry food, hunger in the horse so he gobbles his food, poor condition of teeth, a new, enticing feed introduced too quickly in too-large amounts, a greedy nature.

Too much or too little energy can be due to inappropriate feeding. For instance, too much high-energy feed can certainly make horses very energetic and difficult to control, but too little can make them sluggish and unable to do their work. Many people make the mistake of regarding the 'manger' feed, rather than the hay, as the most important, and so overfeed concentrates. On the other hand, feeding too little concentrate food if the horse is working fairly hard can certainly fail to give him enough energy and enthusiasm for his work. A discussion with your feed company's nutritionist should sort out this problem.

Faulty dentition is a fairly common reason for horses not chewing their feed properly, or not eating enough of it. As people try to economise in the modern economic climate, attention to teeth is often reduced to once a year, when the horse gets his vaccinations (hopefully he still does) and, particularly for horses under four years or over, say 12 of 15 years of age, once a year is not enough, although check with your veterinary practice what they recommend.

Because the upper teeth are set slightly wider than the lower, the inside edges of the lower teeth and the outside edges of the upper teeth can grow too long and sharp, and cut the tongue and cheeks respectively. I shall never forget seeing, many years ago, the skull of a wild horse that appeared to have died of malnutrition. The edges of the upper and lower teeth, as described, had grown inches long and had prevented the horse even closing its mouth and certainly prevented it from eating. This horse was estimated to be only about 10 years old, and I learned that dental troubles were the main cause of death in wild/feral horses, with predation second in countries where they were preyed upon by other animals.

Domestic horses should have their teeth examined and probably rasped down and given other treatment twice a year if young or old (see earlier) or once a year otherwise – or, of course, if they are having trouble such as eating with difficulty, dropping food out of their mouth or leaving much of their feed. This natural propensity of the edges of teeth to become gradually sharp should also, I hope, prompt those of us working them to consider the effect of tight nosebands and harshly-used bits in pressing the cheeks and tongue against the teeth during work. Even if the teeth have smooth edges, pressing soft flesh against hard tooth enamel is bound to be very uncomfortable, and painful if the teeth edges are becoming sharp.

A sharp eye should be kept on all horses to make sure they are not having difficulties in these respects. They should eat easily and freely, not over-manipulating the food in their mouths, dropping it out of their mouths, looking uneasy or troubled when eating or leaving some of a reasonable-sized feed.

The bodyweight of a horse or pony is a good indicator as to his or her diet's suitability, plus the condition of the coat and skin. The fashion is still, today, to over-feed many animals, specifically in what we call 'the western world' where horses mostly work for us in sport or leisure activities and are luxury 'commodities' rather than essential work animals. Animals in the showing world are often criticised for being overweight (not to mention 'over-mounted' by riders too large or heavy for them) and some shows have introduced rules aimed at encouraging owners and producers to present animals of a healthy weight and riders of a suitable weight for their mounts.

Body condition, as well as laminitis, is currently a concern among health care professionals in the horse world. The term 'show condition' has, for decades, meant that horses and ponies have been presented in the showring in an overweight condition, and this has been accepted as 'show condition' by most involved in the showing world, almost having created its own stamp of approval.

I remember visiting, decades ago, a world-famous Arabian stud and meeting some of the most fabled Arabian horses in the world. This was at a time when it was considered good management to have horses in what we would now call an overweight condition. Most of the horses carried too much weight, certainly by today's standards, and the owner and staff chuckled at my tactful remarks about this. They were actually proud of it but were not alone in believing that pads of fat on the horses' backs, behind their shoulders and rounding out their bellies and hindquarters were signs of 'good condition'. Probably the most famous Arab stallion in the world at that time (from another stud) was taken to a prestigious Arab horse show on display (not competing) and was the reason I attended the show as I really wanted to see him. He was elderly but full of life and certainly made his presence felt, snorting and roaring most of the time. His handler, the stud manager, apologised for the horse's having 'lost condition due to his age', but, by today's standards, he was in slim but well-enough covered condition. How times change, in this case for the better.

Those equines kept as pets or companions do not always escape being 'killed with kindness', being allowed sometimes to become unhealthily fat. The quick and easy way of checking a horse's condition, given earlier, of not being able to see his ribs but to feel them quite easily, is a simple, easy guide of healthy weight or condition in any equine. Anything above or below that parameter could indicate an inappropriate weight in the animal concerned which would hopefully be corrected by suitable feeding.

Owners of domestic horses often do not like hearing that feral horses naturally lose weight in winter and put it on again in spring ready for the breeding season. Those ferals unable to maintain their weight through winter will die, reducing the size of the herd. It is true that this may well be nature's apparently cruel but sure fire way of reducing numbers to enable the fittest (as in the most suitable for their environment) to survive, but we do not want our horses to die of cold or starvation! That said, considerably over-feeding horses even in winter can, as we know, lead to various health problems, the most common of which is laminitis, which is not only a spring and summer condition although it is more common then. The aforementioned guideline is still appropriate in winter: if you can easily feel your horse's ribs in winter he would possibly benefit from putting on a little weight but if it is hard to feel them, maybe cut down on the concentrates somewhat.

1.12 CLIPPING

Clipping horses for winter is still done for reasons of 'smartness' but also to prevent excessive sweating in hard-working horses. I have always believed that it is totally unnecessary to clip out or hunter clip any horse, and can actually amount to cruelty if the horse is expected to be standing around in cold weather with little or no protection from his natural coat or from rugs or sheets, and usually with a pulled tail which makes it worse.

It must be obvious that the most inappropriate clip ever is the hunter clip, where hair is only left on the saddle patch and legs in hunters who do spend a considerable amount of time standing around during the day. Horses naturally stand with their tails to the wind and weather and pulled tails offer them no protection in this regard. The hunter clip is still widely used for smartness and is a clear indication of the owner's higher regard for appearance than for their horse's well-being. The compromise is the

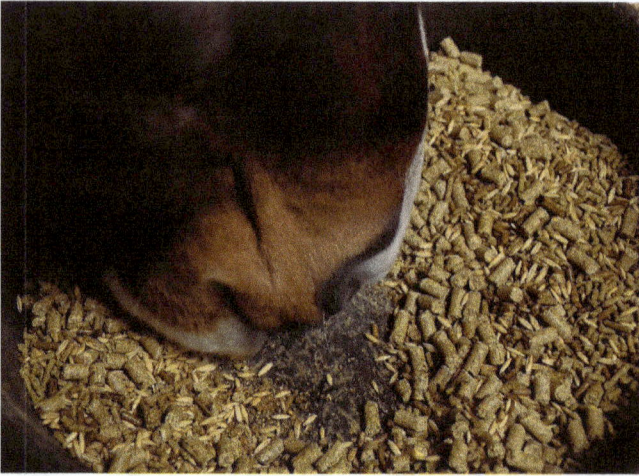

Figure 1.1 Concentrate feeds such as grains (oats, barley, etc.) and cubes or horse nuts should not be regarded as a horse's staple diet. Their role is to add an extra dimension (possibly under specialist supervision) for horses working hard or in poor condition due to incorrect or insufficient feeding.
Source: (Shutterstock ID: 2289982671)

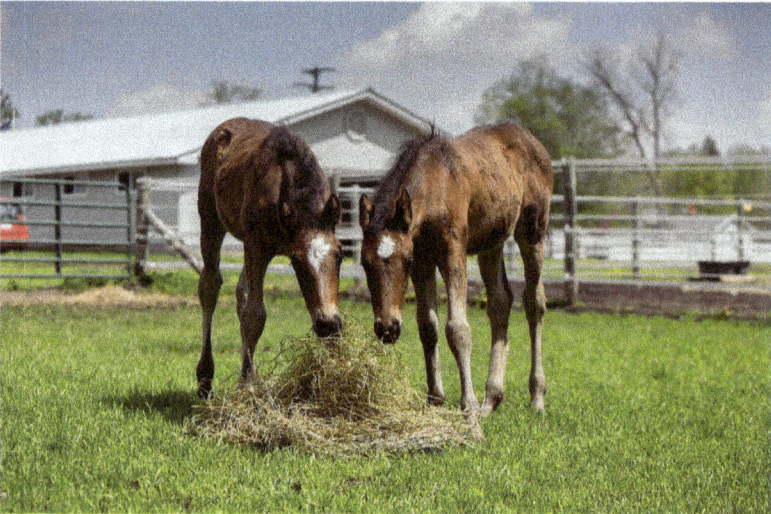

Figure 1.2 The most important feed for most horses is the best quality hay. This means clean (not dusty or mouldy), feeling springy to the feel ('well made') and of appropriate feeding value (nutrient content) for the circumstances of and physical demands on the horse, such as light or harder work, breeding, convalescing and so on.
Source: (Shutterstock ID: 327125384)

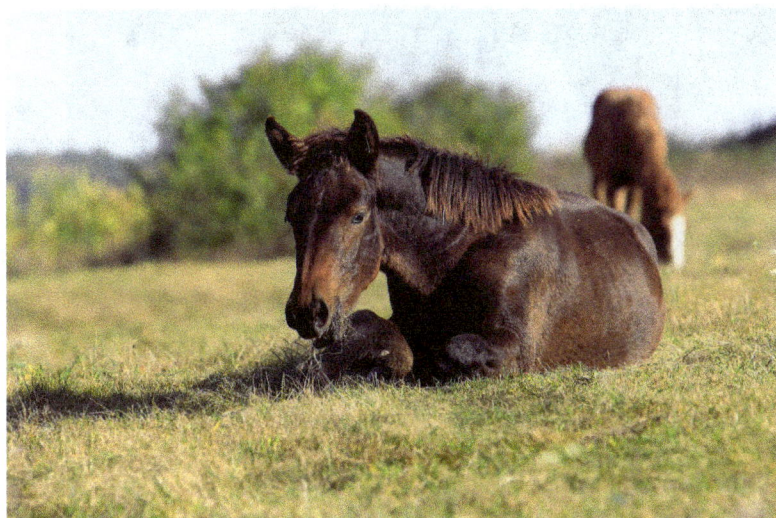

Figure 1.3 There's nothing like having a snack while you're resting.
Source: (Shutterstock ID: 38512108)

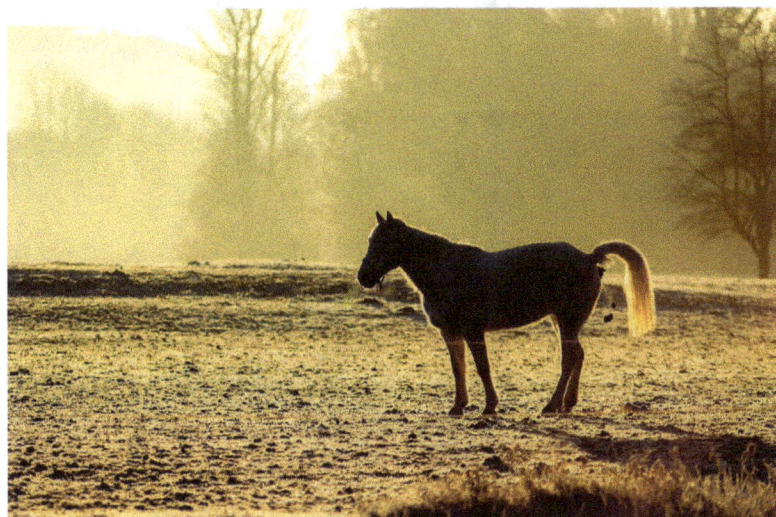

Figure 1.4 Horse manure should be picked up as often as is reasonably possible to avoid its contaminating the grassland with its smell and taste. Ideally, droppings should be removed within two hours to avoid this happening and so discouraging horses from eating nearby. If they are left much longer, the horses designate the surrounding area as a lavatory area, refuse to graze there and so the grass grows long and becomes unpalatable, whereas their eating areas away from the droppings may be over-grazed.
Source: (Shutterstock ID: 1321892546)

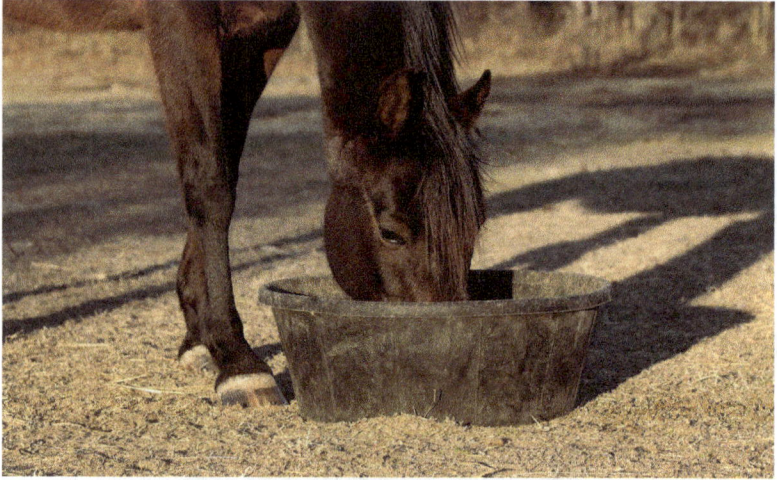

Figure 1.5 Ideally, free-standing bowls like this should be avoided for feeding horses outdoors as they are often tipped over by the horse and much of the feed wasted in the grassland. However, rubber, like this one, is much safer than metal.
Source: (Shutterstock ID: 2075980789)

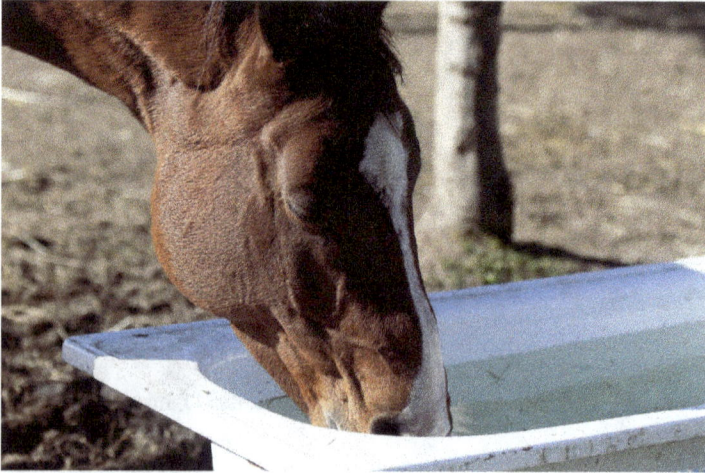

Figure 1.6 Old baths are often used as drinking troughs for outdoor horses. If they have rolled tops, the sharp edges can easily injure horses' knees if they stamp their forelegs while drinking, as is fairly common. Whatever container is used, it should be checked for any points and edges that could potentially injure the horses.
Source: (Shutterstock ID: 2076662956)

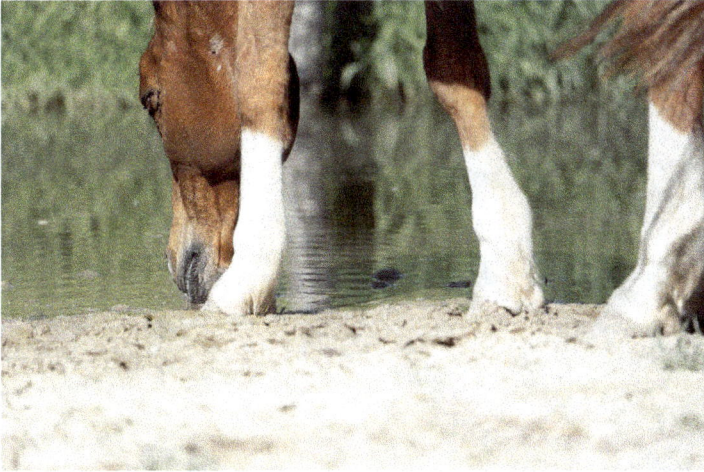

Figure 1.7 Drinking from ground level is the natural position for horses. The water is forced up the oesophagus by muscular contractions and then passes down into the stomach. Many horses need to splay their legs so that they can get their mouths down far enough to reach the water. We should always check that a horse can easily reach and drink water if his source is at ground level so that he is not deprived of enough water to satisfy himself. Where necessary, water should be provided in safe containers that allow horses to reach the water easily and safely: they obviously need to be kept clean and topped up.
Source: (Shutterstock ID: 2468193849)

blanket clip in which the hair is left on the horse's back and, crucially, his sides and hind-quarters, which at least gives him *some* protection. An even kinder clip would be a high trace clip without the head, in which hair is also left on the upper shoulders and tapered up the neck to behind the horse's ears. And if we're talking of kindness, it would be in the horse's favour to leave his tail full on the dock and banged across the bottom, racehorse-style.

1.13 FORAGING

Foraging, that is hunting out, smelling and selecting food occupies most of the time of horses out in fairly natural conditions – grazing grasses and browsing leaves. At liberty, they do this for most of their 24 hours. Horses need roughly four to six hours sleep out of the 24 which leaves them the many hours needed to acquire and digest their food. They are made this way and need to be able to do it. However, very many domesticated

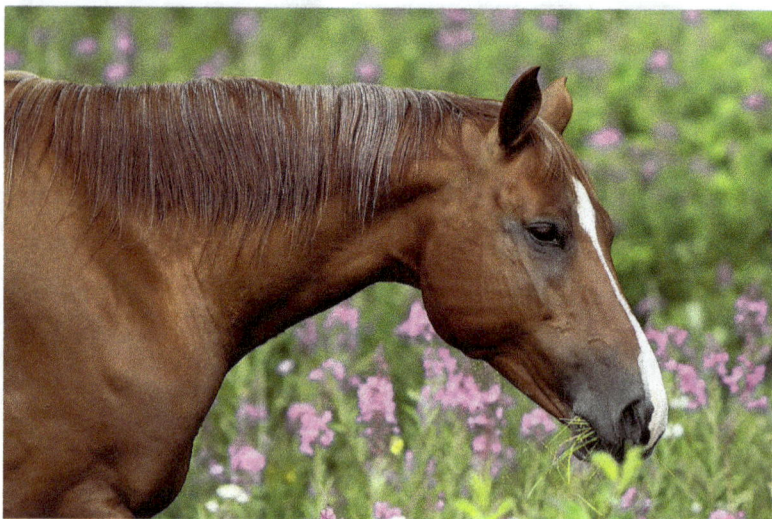

Figure 1.8 Although most horses love 'domestic' foods being given to them, other growing plants need to be checked out for identity and whether or not they are poisonous. Horses do not seem to naturally avoid toxic plants.

Source: (Shutterstock ID: 109819766)

horses do not have the opportunity to practice this essential occupation, either because they are not turned out on grass or, when stabled, are not given enough food (mainly as in appropriate hay or haylage) to do so.

When conditions make it impossible to turn out horses on grass they are often turned out together on a surfaced or simply earth enclosure for a sense of freedom and exercise and haynets or other containers for hay or haylage made available for them. This is a fair alternative for them and means that they can still experience freedom and the company of their friends and have food available during their turnout time. It is good to provide different types of hay for them around the enclosure, so giving them some of the sense of variety they would experience in a grass area.

If you wander around among horses grazing naturally, in company, on grazing that is adequate to plentiful, and perhaps with trees and shrubs available as well, you cannot miss the atmosphere of all's being right with their world. The air of relaxation, satisfaction and sheer enjoyment is palpable. We should remember that their mental health as well as their physical well-being is crucial to their overall welfare. Anything that can promote it should be regarded as their right and not, as is so often

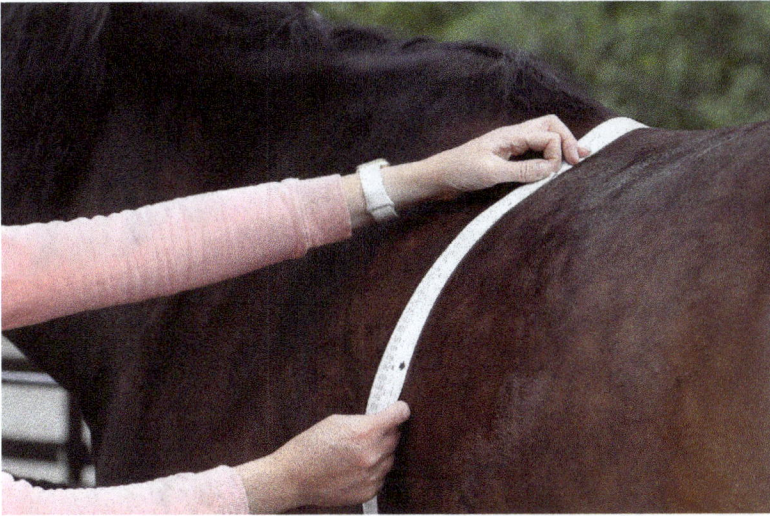

Figure 1.9 Buying your own weigh-tape and learning how to use it correctly is very helpful in monitoring your horse's bodyweight. The tape should be flat, straight and passed around the horse's trunk behind the withers. A weekly weighing like this should be included in your regular health check. Other pointers such as general demeanour, body temperature, condition of skin and coat, soundness and breathing should, with advantage, be checked and recorded every week as a matter of course. Everyone, though, should be constantly on the lookout for changes in a horse's condition or behaviour on a daily basis.
Source: (Shutterstock ID: 2327476813)

the case, regarded as a treat. Being with friends enjoying the facility of sorting out food as evolution created them to live should be allowed and encouraged as much as possible.

There is still a belief in some quarters of the horse world that bulky feeds like hay and roots should be limited so that horses can work better. It is true that horses should not be worked straight after they have been eating hay for some time or a moderate to large manger feed, but most horses' work periods comprise a relatively small part of their day. If the nutrient content and level of their feed is carefully watched in accordance with their work, there is no reason to deny horses anything that helps them to be happy, settled, confident in their daily lives that their needs are met, and to keep them in appropriate condition for whatever type of work they do. Like humans, horses and other animals can develop various physical and mental disorders from experiencing any level of

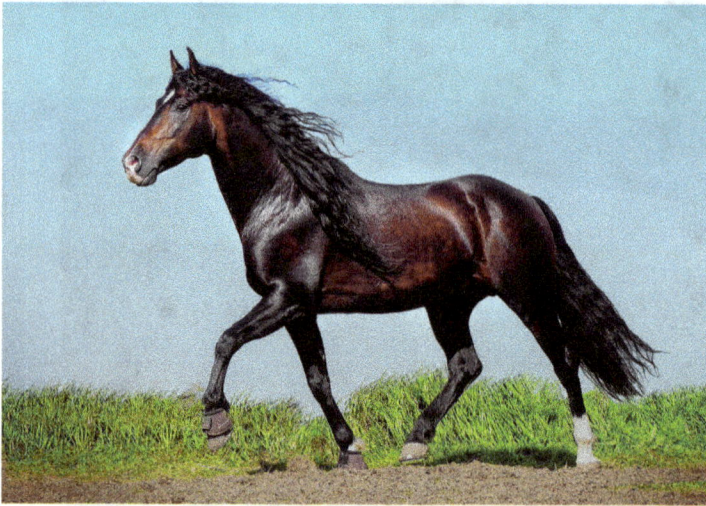

Figure 1.10 A beautiful horse in splendid condition, oozing good health and well-being.

Source: (Shutterstock ID: 78394738)

discontentment, particularly when it is a regular part of their lives. Stress can be a killer and a trigger for many disorders in humans and animals living lives inappropriate for them. In horses, we find many abnormal behaviours, formerly called 'stable vices' as though the horse were misbehaving rather than being mis-managed, but today they are known more correctly as stereotypical behaviours. There are various triggers for these, but hunger is a significant one on yards where it is still believed that 'too much' hay prevents horses working well or that concentrate feeds are more important than bulky roughage feeds, as mentioned earlier. Timing feed in working horses is explained earlier. With expert help from a vet and/or equine nutritionist, it is perfectly possible to give a horse the type of diet he needs for comfort and satisfaction while feeding him appropriately for both work and health.

Horses evolved to be in company, to roam and to eat for most of their 24 hours and the nearer we can get to this situation in a domestic life, whether our horses are working or not, the happier and healthier they will be.

Two

It's no secret and we all know it – horses are creatures of wide, open spaces and live naturally in herds. Compare that with the scene on almost any equestrian yard – one or many rows of individual loose boxes, indoor or outdoor, with, hopefully, turn-out areas on grass or surfaced areas, or at least a covered or indoor area where horses can enjoy some freedom and close, tactile company.

The fact that horses live apparently contented lives in such seemingly inappropriate environments is a tribute to their versatility. On well-managed yards (and the term 'yard', as we know, means 'equestrian accommodation facility'), horses and ponies get used to their routine. They know when they usually get turned out with friends, when they will be fed, perhaps when they will be exercised or worked, groomed and so on. They also know when a day is 'different', such as when they are going off the yard in transport perhaps to some show or other event, when the farrier or vet has arrived, what time various daily events occur such as feeding, turnout, grooming, disappearance of all humans at night and so on.

If equines are fairly treated, routined, correctly fed, bedded down, turned out on acceptable surfaces with or without grass (and, in the latter case, hopefully hay or haylage supplied in various containers), exercised perhaps in a school or out on a hack and so on, it is amazing, given the type of animal they are, that they do adapt to a horse-friendly routine with reasonable equanimity. They feel safe, they have friends and perhaps family, they come to know, I am sure, that when they are injured or ill they will be cared for even if veterinary attentions are somewhat uncomfortable, and they generally feel an undercurrent of confidence that all is reasonably well with their world.

2.1 EQUINE SOCIETY AND RELATIONSHIPS

Horses in natural, wild or feral conditions, live in family groups. Contrary to popular opinion, the stallion is only a lodger among the mares and

DOI: 10.1201/9781003396376-3

youngsters, the true leader usually being an older, experienced mare. The process is that young colts obviously grow up and usually start trying it on with mares young and old in their family group but are usually put firmly in their place, especially by senior mares. They will be the offspring of the current stallion or the one before. Whatever – once they show signs of puberty the current stallion, if still fit and well, ousts bolshi young colts from the herd, which is why, in appropriate areas, there are bands of young entires living free, possibly missing their family, but naturally wanting to create their own family or fight for and take over an existing herd. Sometimes, instead, they may succeed in stealing a young filly or two from an existing herd and start their own family that way. A mature herd stallion is a formidable foe unless he is on the decline due to age, sickness or injury.

In domestic conditions things are not allowed to work that way. Young entire horses will not get the chance to mate with the females as they will be separated at puberty. If, though, they are on a stud, an outstanding colt may be kept as a stallion.

In feral conditions, although the herd stallion, once accepted by the mature mares, can form close relationships with his mares and offspring, it is the mares who are the nucleus of the herd. Although stallions may be displaced by younger ones, this does not happen with mares, who usually stay with the herd even if they have no offspring in a particular year or are past breeding. Often older mares, and stallions if they have not been challenged, stay with the herd but tend to graze on the outskirts of it, not getting involved with the daily socialising of the others. In my previous book to this one, *Partnering Your Horse*, I told the true story of one such elderly mare the others largely ignored but who took charge and saw off a young bullock who broke into their field, driving him back to the break in the fence and standing guard until the fence was mended. Many older mares may seem to us to be on the fringes of herd society but may well not be considered so by the other horses. An old mare of mine was certainly the boss, when necessary, of all the other horses in the field when disputes arose, and I have known this to be so in many cases. Older horses are also often allowed the pick of the grazing and water. Youngsters might even go to them for protection when there is trouble.

In domestic conditions, horses are rarely allowed to choose their own friends. Horses' kicks and bites are very dangerous, a kick being easily able to break the leg of a human or another horse. Bites, too, can be very damaging. Horses' relationships can be very close with each other, and they need friends and possibly family members just as much as humans and other animals do. It is sad that, being prone to being bought and sold as they are for different purposes, their friendships are often destroyed when they are parted. This can cause them just as much sadness and mental trauma as it can for us.

I certainly disagree with the attitude that horses should not be allowed to form close friendships as this will cause trouble when they are separated for work. There is no need to worry about this in a correctly managed and well-routined horse or horses. They can and, I believe, should be stabled with or next to each other because, remember, their non-working time is much greater than their time working for us. The way to get two closely attached horses to get used to working or being handled individually, maybe not even with their friend visible, is to tackle it very gradually, mixing them with other friendly horses for, say, hacking, or manège work for, initially, short periods, and gradually over weeks working and dealing with them separately. They get to know that they will be reunited with their friends before long. This can also be done with short trips travelling and, of course, can result in the two horses attending different events without their soul-mate, knowing that they will be reunited.

When you are faced with the opposite situation of a horse being stabled next to, or even near, a horse with whom he does not get on, being either the aggressor or the underling, it is sensible and correct management to stable them as far as possible away from each other. The attitude of 'well, they'll just have to get used to it' is totally inappropriate, bad horse management which can actually result in damaged physical and even mental health in the horse on the receiving end of the other's dislike or aggression.

Situations like this do cause problems on, for example, livery yards or other establishments where, for instance, a horse may have been sent for training. There may be limited accommodation and it may not be possible to change your horse's box. Unfortunately, this can only be dealt with in situ when you find out there is a problem.

As for horses' relationships with humans, there is a good deal of debate on this issue. It has to be admitted that there are plenty of people in the horse world internationally who use horses for money or prestige and should not really be called horsemen or women. The way to a horse's heart and head is through correct training and management, including handling and riding, and I have covered this in detail in my books *Fine Riding* and *Partnering Your Horse*. Basically, real classical riding combined with the correct application of Equitation Science, in which there have been great discoveries in the past 20 or so years, are the way to go.

2.2 EXPLAINING EQUITATION SCIENCE

One of the most common mistakes we make with horses is to believe, rather naturally, that they think like we do – but they don't. Equitation Science is based on *equine learning theory* – training horses according to how they really think and learn. It uses methods of training, working, handling and managing horses shown by modern scientific evidence to be humane and effective, and easily understandable and beneficial to horses, with their equine brains.

The objective of the best domestic horse care and management is to make sure our horses have whatever they want and need to be healthy and happy (disregarding the opinion still held in some quarters that horses cannot be proven to experience happiness!).

We all know that horses evolved as creatures of wide, open spaces, living in mainly family herds, and grazing many varied species of grasses and other plants, plus browsing on leaves from trees and shrubs. We also know that in most parts of the world domestic horses' freedom is greatly curtailed, as is their contact with other horses or ponies and also their access to foraging – the searching for, sorting and eating fibrous food for roughly 16 hours a day.

The International Society for Equitation Science (www. equitationscience.com) has earmarked that a lifestyle of Friends, Freedom and Foraging is the most important to horses themselves, the essential trio of qualities in their lives that is in general the most essential and which occupies far more of their time than we do. I cannot remember a time in my fairly long life when there was so much study, research and deep interest in horses in the academic and scientific communities – their lives, their psychology and physiology, how they think and learn which is different from how we have assumed, what they like, dislike and fear, and what they must have in order to be healthy and happy. The above Three F's, as they are known, are an excellent basis for reliably good horse care and management.

2.3 FRIENDS

As herd animals, horses by nature rely on others for daily companionship and friendship, but our idea of horses' need for company is often not the same as theirs. We have been seeing horses in rows of separate stables for so many generations, indeed thousands of years, that it seems to have almost become second nature for us to keep them in that way. Yet the only worse way, in most cases, is to keep a horse in a stable alone, without another horse in sight or within scenting and hearing distance, let alone the ability to touch each other.

(There are rare examples of horses who genuinely do not like others. Some, also, get on when at liberty but not when stabled next to each other and vice versa. There may be various reasons for these situations and an expert, such as a member of the Association of Pet Behaviour Counsellors (www.apbc.org.uk), the word 'pet' here also covering horses, may well be able to offer rehabilitation to such horses and advice for their owners.

One reason for the successful survival of the equine species is its adaptability. If horses are given adequate freedom – several hours a day depending on the weather and climate – they are often quite happy and look forward to coming in to a clean, ample bed, fresh water, sweet hay or haylage and perhaps some other, more concentrated feed and succulents in the manger. They are particularly keen to come in for shelter during adverse weather and environmental conditions (such as insects) at any time of year, especially if their outdoor accommodation lacks effective shelter facilities. Man-made shelter offers far better protection from insects than trees, which positively attract flies.

Stabling in itself is not 'a bad thing': it is the *type* of stabling that has been receiving much more attention worldwide in recent years, with studies monitoring horses' activities when in different designs of stabling, how long they spend eating, drinking, lying down, sleeping, dozing standing up, self-grooming, looking out onto the yard and so on. This work has enabled researchers to pinpoint what elements of domestic life really make horses happier, calmer, healthier and generally feeling content and secure (hence the Three F's), and the most important to the horses has been found to be friendly company of their own kind – and not just on an occasional basis.

Horses' adaptability enables them to cope with being stabled to some extent, but, not surprisingly, it has been found that horses are calmer, with lower heart rates and fewer 'stress hormones' but more 'happy hormones' circulating in their bodies when they are in stables that give as much space, variety and interest as possible and, most particularly, when they are able to touch friendly, neighbouring horses. The points most valued by the horses have been confirmed to be the ability to touch, smell and, if possible, groom with friends in neighbouring stables. This, of course, goes directly against the old rule that horses must not be allowed to touch each other in stables as it might promote fighting. The most important word to remember in this important updating of advice is 'friendly'.

Also valued are additional comforts such as a small yard leading from each individual box where they and their (friendly) neighbours can come and go as they like and socialise, more than one outlook to the outside, more than one supply of different forage (hay or haylage) to provide variety which, however, can never contain the number of species available in natural foraging.

It is sad to note that more and more modern owners are reluctant to let their horses do what is most important to them – be really with their friends. Being able just to see other horses when stabled is no longer regarded as enough, particularly for horses who are kept in a conventional, fairly 'sterile', basic loose box for long periods of time, with only an hour or two of freedom daily. Lines of stables in which horses may be able to only see each other without any other kind of meaningful (to them) contact advantageously could be adapted to make possible the aforementioned sorts of contact and activities, for the horses' better well-being and health.

Friendships should be encouraged whether the horses are in or out and, of course, known hostile horses kept separate, as mentioned earlier, again both in and out. Stable neighbours should be friends or, at least, neutral in their attitudes to each other. The modern practice (in the UK at least) of using taped-off, 'postage-stamp'-sized areas of ground in which horses can see each other, sniff over the usually-electrified tape but not socialise naturally or sufficiently, not to mention graze adequately, have been described in one study as causing mental cruelty similar to a carrot on a stick. Point taken. It is also very bad for the land.

Settled groups of known friends have an extremely low level of 'turnout injuries' because there is no need for antagonism. Horses in a correctly chosen and socialised group do not habitually kick, bite and harass each other. The groups do not have to be identical each time horses are put out, but they should all get to know each other very well and be together with mostly the same individuals, with newcomers introduced gradually and carefully. Hacking together, working in the school together or being led out to graze together are all acceptable and safe ways of socialising horses with each other. Follow up by turning out the newcomer with one horse he or she seems to have taken to, and take it from there.

2.4 FREEDOM

Freedom is, of course, the quality we most associate with a natural style of life for horses.

If horses are turned loose together so they are absolutely free to mutually groom, wander together often with shoulders touching while grazing, play together, lie down together, shelter together, generally communicate in Equus together, and so on, and also have adequate occupation, exploration and food (all of which foraging involves), they have nearly all they could want.

Friendly horses and/or ponies kept communally in covered yards, particularly with a good view outside, and especially in a large shelter open to a fenced, surfaced area outside, also display contentment, calmness, happiness and security – enviable states for all of us. Long racks of hay and haylage at chest height in the shelter are an appropriate and quick way of providing food and foraging, and drinkers or a trough, kept clean, are also needed.

Of course, the smaller the area allocated to the horses the more meticulous we need to be over poo-picking. Horses choose not to graze within a metre of equine droppings, whether their own or those of other equines. Unfortunately, if fresh droppings are not picked up within ten to 30 minutes of being deposited, they sour the land with a lasting smell distasteful to horses, and collection at this frequency is impractical. In a covered, surfaced yard or shelter with open yard, they can be picked up quite frequently but not in acres of grassland.

(Following on from the horses when they move on to a different field as in a good rotation system would, ideally, be a herd of cattle which actually sweeten the land rather than sour it – and they do not mind grazing near equine droppings, so an even growth of grass and soil health are maintained.)

Horses' urinating and dunging practices of creating 'lavatory areas' not used for grazing is the reason for the development in their paddocks of 'roughs' for droppings and urine which grow long, unpalatable grass, and 'lawns' of clean areas which can become overgrazed. (This grazing pattern is one reason farmers do not like horses grazing their land, another being that galloping, playing horses do a lot of damage to damp or wet turf.) If you, or your livery yard, are in the fortunate position of having enough land to rotate every few weeks, you can adopt the method devised by Dr Marytavy Archer at the former Equine Research Station in Newmarket back in, I think, the late 1960s or '70s.

First, in a simple rota of three paddocks, cattle are put on one paddock to eat off the long grass as they cannot graze short grass due to having no upper incisors, or front teeth, so grass has to be long enough for them to be able to tear it off with their tongues. They also sweeten the pasture with their droppings. Cattle and horses do not object to each other's droppings and urine. When the cattle move to paddock 2 after a few weeks, the horses go on to paddock 1 and have plenty of keep left for them by the cattle, who have grazed down the roughs the horses won't graze and disguised the smell of the horses' previous droppings with their own, deposited randomly on the paddock, so fertilising the lawns as well, and making the roughs acceptable to the horses. Then, the cattle move to paddock 3, the horses follow them to paddock 2, then the first paddock is cleared of any remaining horse droppings and rested, and maybe treated, until it has grown enough to provide grazing for the cattle again.

In this way, horses and cattle do each other and the land a big favour. Land treatments, essential to keep land in good heart and the grass sweet, can be fitted in as required – such as removal of remaining horse droppings (scattering them makes the contamination worse), harrowing not least to spread the cattle droppings, fertilising, removing poisonous growing things and so on, although the latter should be a constant activity.

If you do not have enough land for this, seriously consider mixed grazing with dehorned cattle and horses using two paddocks. Even small paddocks can be managed well in this way, say two horses and two or three cattle. Check with your vet about cattle diseases and medications that could possibly be passed on from the cattle. Obviously, horned cattle are not suitable. Parasites in cattle droppings will not adversely affect the horses' health. (Sheep, incidentally, are not so helpful as cattle because they graze even shorter than horses and seem to spend a lot of time asleep, anyway!)

With schemes like the aforementioned, you can provide your horses with what they need, or even create a 'paddock paradise' arrangement to keep them moving around – tracks between different paddocks which are kept open or locked on a rota basis. The animals will feel secure, content, healthy and happy. It would be good if more farmers with a diversified livery enterprise would create such a facility or even just the rota, for the benefit of all concerned.

2.5 FORAGING

Horses evolved to spend roughly two-thirds of their time foraging for food, as mentioned. Two-thirds. That's a long time, but it is how they are made and extensive foraging is an in-built need for them. It's not that they are greedy: they just don't have a choice. This means that when that time is reduced because horses are on a human-devised diet and regime, such as high-concentrate requirements for hard-working horses, which usually results in reduced fibre provision, they can suffer from digestive problems ranging from slight discomfort to serious ones like colic and ulcers mainly in the stomach but also in other parts of the digestive system.

This is because the horse evolved as a fairly continuous eater, producing digestive acid all the time. When eating naturally for most of the time, lightly grazing and browsing, and/or with a mainly *ad lib* supply of hay or haylage, this acid is put to good use, but when we restrict their diet to less bulky fibre and, perhaps, more concentrate feed, the horses' nutrient needs are met in a much shorter time, the acid is not used and injures the delicate lining of the digestive system. Digestive system ulcers in horses are difficult and expensive to treat for us and very painful for the horse, so we need to devise appropriate diets that provide correct nutrients with sufficient feed to cope with the acid. Ulcers form quickly: *it is recommended widely by veterinarians and equine nutritionists that horses are not left for more than four hours without food, to help prevent ulceration.*

As for not feeding them before working, it is advised that horses due to work hard and/or fast should be given, say, a double handful of fibre feed such as chopped hay, haylage or a bagged fibre feed, half an hour before starting work. This will help to stop acid in the horse's stomach splashing up onto the stomach walls and triggering ulcers.

2.6 BOREDOM

We should not overlook the most important occupational value to horses of eating for most of the time. They didn't evolve to tolerate boredom and do not experience it in natural conditions. The combination of an unsuitable man-made diet made worse by over-confinement can result in many hours with nothing to do (bearing in mind that horses only sleep for about four to six hours and in short snatches) and positively invites the development of stereotypies (formerly called 'stable vices' as though the horse were doing something wrong as opposed to trying to relieve his discomfort) and other psychological and physical upsets – seriously inappropriate management for an animal like a horse.

Today, equine nutrition is a more advanced science than ever before, and it is quite possible to create feeds and, indeed, grassland seed mixes of the appropriate energy and nutrient content for a horse's lifestyle while catering for his evolutionary needs and health requirements. Every decent equine feed firm will have a free helpline to a qualified nutritionist who can help you come up with a suitable diet for your horse as an individual, his work, if any, and his lifestyle including access to grazing and browsing. It is possible to have hay and haylage analysed, and it is advised because of their importance to the horse's digestive comfort and health: the concentrate or 'manger' feed can then be chosen to provide any missing nutrients or energy needs.

The traditional grasses found to be good for hard-working and stud blood horses — mostly ryegrass and timothy — are too 'rich' for most horses except racing bloodstock, mainly Thoroughbreds. In some equines, ryegrass and timothy have also been found to cause skin problems originally thought to be sweet itch. Cattle pastures, too, are often meant for milk-producing cows rather than less demanding beef cattle, and again are too nutritious for most horses and certainly ponies and cross-breds. Many warmbloods, too, cannot take such diets. When farms are diversified for equestrian businesses, land is rarely reseeded to suit horses rather than cattle, so horse owners' only option is to reduce the time spent out grazing, which may not be best for the horses.

I feel it is time we reassessed our traditional views of entire diets for our equines, for the sake of their health and — that word again — happiness. We need diets to keep them in good health for their lifestyles while allowing them to explore, find and experience many different tastes — in practice, to forage and satisfy their hunger and curiosity as nature intended, whether indoors or out.

2.7 EATING LIKE HORSES

The ideal diet, of course, would provide what is needed purely from hay and haylage, so that we could get away from the traditional human-style system of feeding a few separate 'meals' throughout the 24 hours and regarding them as the horse's main food, with hay/haylage as only a back-up. In fact, it should be the other way round.

Bagged fibrous feeds are readily available in different nutrient and energy contents, reducing the need for concentrates, but they are not cheap. However, horses do like them and they can be made even more attractive by the addition of succulents such as sugar beet pulp or thinly sliced apples or carrots (horses can choke on chunks). Horses often like to have a whole turnip or swede left in their manger to chomp on.

The more horse-appropriate we can make our horses' diets and lives, the happier and healthier they will be.

2.8 THE OUTDOOR LIFE, PROS AND CONS

There is no doubt that horses evolved as animals for an outdoor life, their characteristics evolving according to their 'home' climate. Basically, in cold climates horses and ponies evolved with thicker skins and longer, coarser coats than those that evolved in hot climates, which produce thinner skins and finer, shorter coats. The former features offer some heat-retaining protection against the cold climate whereas the latter enables horses to shed heat easier in warm to hot climates.

Horses do not make dens, they do not hibernate, and they are not solitary. They live normally in herds, they have a year-round lifestyle and they spend most of their time grazing in the open, although also browsing leaves from trees and shrubs. They evolved long necks and heads which makes browsing easier but also enables them to reach down to the ground from those long legs which evolved for galloping away from predators.

The horse's early ancestors used to have four toes on their front feet and three on the back ones whereas, of course, this number has, through evolution, dwindled down to one in today's whole equine family (horses and ponies, asses or donkeys and the various types of zebra), who have only one, the only animals in the world to have this single digit – equivalent to our middle finger and toe. It is sometimes said that this is why they are so fast, but the fastest land animal in the world, the cheetah, a cat, has, of course, multiple toes. Domestic cats, interestingly, have been seen to keep up easily with horses galloping (not just cantering) in their paddocks.

Fast cats have two moments of suspension in the air per stride which means their stride has less of the slowing-down effect caused by contact with the ground. Horses have only one – after the leading leg has landed. When the stride starts again with a hind foot, all four feet hit the ground in succession, the gallop being a four-beat gait. The horse may start its stride in gallop with, say, the left hind followed by the right hind, then the left fore and finishing by 'leading' with the right fore. In cheetahs, for example, one hind foot hits the ground to start the stride, as in horses, followed by the second hind foot. However, instead of the first forefoot then landing there is a moment of suspension in the air before the first forefoot lands, followed by the second ('leading' foot or leg), and then there is another moment of suspension before the hind feet start the next stride. This permits greater speed than possessed by an animal with only one moment of suspension. The top speed of a cheetah is about 69 to 75 miles per hour whereas the top speed of a Thoroughbred racehorse has been clocked at 44 mph. American Quarter Horses, without a rider, can run at 55 mph over short distances but the average galloping speed of an 'ordinary' horse is about 25 mph. Cheetahs, however, rarely tackle prey as large as an equine, say, a zebra, as they themselves are smaller, much lighter and not so strong as equines.

The outside walls of horse's feet are fully protected by hard horn which grows continuously, as we all know, like our much weaker fingernails. The feet have very sensitive tissue on the inside of the hoof walls which is what becomes inflamed and extremely painful in the increasingly common disease (in the UK) we know as laminitis. The ground surface of the hoof is more sensitive than the wall, comprising the slightly arched, horny sole and the softer frog running down the middle of the foot from the heels. Feral horses wear their hooves down surprisingly evenly but domestic ones regularly need the skilled care, trimming and balancing of a good farrier, whether or not they wear metal shoes.

Time was when the farrier would also attend to horses' teeth, but today we have specially trained equine dentists for this vital job. The teeth of young and old domestic horses and ponies need attention twice a year on average, age groups in between usually managing on once a year.

Horses' coats change twice a year in spring and autumn, from a thinner but still protective one in summer to a thicker, longer one for warmth in winter. Unfortunately, their winter coats do not entirely protect them from heavy, prolonged rain, but they certainly help while unfortunately sometimes providing a home for skin parasites which not only cause constant irritation but can also enable skin infections to develop and also blood loss from the insects sucking the horses' blood. Horses' manes, forelocks and tails help with the protection from both winter weather and summer sun, especially those animals who develop double-sided manes, much to the possible annoyance of their human owners. It is, of course, natural for the tail to consist of long hair from the dock downwards and horses soon learn to use this excellent protection to stand with their hindquarters to the prevailing wind and weather.

Domestic horses mostly have their coats clipped to some extent and their forelocks, manes and tail hair trimmed or removed in various ways by us humans. There is a widespread idea that this 'smartens' up a horse just for appearance sake or because the horse is shown in appropriate classes. I am among those who believe in as little interference as possible commensurate with comfort and reason.

Clipping the coat has been done with various machines for a few hundred years. I well remember the hand-operated clipping machine used on the horses and ponies at the excellent, classical riding school at which I first learned to ride. It had a large wheel turned by hand which worked the clipper blades, I cannot remember how, and we children had to take it in turns to turn it when clipping time came in the autumn. It was such hard work we couldn't maintain the effort for long! (As well as our paid-for lessons, we were expected to attend and help around the yard with the stable work for free. This gave us valuable experience of the various jobs, and the hard work, involved in not only looking after the horses and ponies but also generally running a yard and understanding horses and their needs.)

Clipping does have a purpose, and is not merely for so-called smartness. If a horse is working fairly hard, constant and possibly heavy sweating is, as you can imagine, energy-draining and can severely chill the horse as he is cooling down, particularly if his attendant does not take the trouble to rug him up with appropriate anti-sweat clothing and walk him until he has cooled down, usually allowing several sips of water during pauses. I do believe, though, that a horse should be clipped as little as is commensurate with his level of physical exertion. To clip a horse like a hunter 'all out' (all the hair removed) is, in my view, cruel because hunters spend a good amount of time, possibly steaming after galloping, standing around in cold winter weather. This is appallingly bad welfare care. A traditional hunter clip leaves on a patch of hair for the saddle and the hair on the legs, while probably trimming the fetlock hair. This sort of clip might provide some degree of smartness but is not horse-friendly, in my view.

Excellent compromises are the trace and the 'chaser' clip, which leave hair on the upper part of the body, with the head hair being removed in the 'chaser' ('steeplechaser') clip. There is also the useful blanket clip in which the hair is removed from the head, neck, breast, shoulders and belly, but left on elsewhere. In other words, if you put a blanket on the horse from the withers backwards, that is the area (and the legs) on which the hair is kept, so basically only the forehand and belly are clipped.

I much prefer full tail hair left on the dock of any horse or pony for year-round protection. The dock hair can be temporarily plaited/braided for appearance's sake, when required, but not too tightly as this can cause pain. As the tail is also crucial for removing insects from the rear half of the horse, the tail hair should not be over-shortened either: mid-hind-canon length seems suitable for most horses and ponies. My favourite style of tail hair for any working horse or pony is what is generally called 'the racehorse tail' in which the hair is left full at the top and banged (cut level) across the bottom to about mid-canon length. If not working, of course still leave the dock hair and let the rest of it grow to protect against weather and insects.

Clipping the lower legs is also often done for smartness and ease of cleaning. Arguments vary as to whether or not to clip legs. The hair's purpose is to protect the legs from wet conditions, but there is no doubt that serious skin problems, commonly known as 'mud fever', can occur under all this hair if the wet and mud penetrate it to the skin. It is necessary to keep a close eye on the skin under these 'feathers', as they are called, and promptly treat any skin problems. If the hair is removed, the natural protection is removed, but it does enable the legs to be kept clean and wet mud more easily removed, the usual advice being to allow it to dry and then brush it off rather than washing it off, which removes more of the skin's natural protective oils. As mentioned later, cattle udder cream is a good preventative for mud fever.

2.9 FENCING

Keeping horses where we want them and allowing them freedom as well necessitates fencing of some kind. Unfortunately, with the now-common diversification of some farms to at least partial livery facilities for horses, barbed wire fencing around horse paddocks is not unknown but should be avoided like the plague by any caring owner. I feel that it is one of the worse inventions of modern life so far as keeping animals is concerned. Cattle may be quieter than horses, but I have still seen some awful injuries to them from barbed wire. Horses, prone as they are to playing, cavorting and galloping around (which is partly why we turn them out to give them this opportunity) should *never* be put near barbed wire, whether it is surrounding a paddock, lining a riding track or wherever. It is not a question, as one farmer put it to me, that once they have an altercation with a barbed wire fence they won't go near it again. Horses do not rationalise or have the same logic abilities as we do and when in a panic or over-excited, either in a good or bad way, they do not think about the danger of the fence. Even plain wire is far from ideal for horses. It is not easily visible and horses can get the wire strands between the heels of their shoes and their hooves, with disastrous consequences.

Fencing for horses has come a long way from the still-excellent wooden posts and rails. Posts and rails themselves are often erected incorrectly. The rails should be on the *inside* of the paddocks so that horses cantering along the fence-line will not injure their shoulders on the posts, even if the posts are round which they usually are not. Also, the top rail should be fixed right to the tops of the posts so that any horse jumping out, as they sometimes do, will not sustain a bad injury to his belly on the top of the post, especially a square post with a flat top and, of course, corners.

Strong synthetic materials are now often used for fencing and these construction factors should be followed when using them, too. As for the distance between rails and the height of the fencing, any fencing should be at least the height of the horses' withers to discourage jumping out, but this is often far from the case. For breeding stock, the lower rail should be low enough to prevent a foal rolling through the gap and ending up, panicking, on the wrong side of the fence from his dam. There can be one, two or, rarely, three additional rails in between the top and bottom rails, depending on whether the paddock is for ponies or large horses.

It should be remembered that stallions smelling a mare in season, even on the wind blowing towards him, can fairly easily jump out over a normal-height fence to offer the mare his services, which is the main reason that special stallion paddock fencing is often as high as the horses' heads, and may be close boarded as well. However, it is not unknown for horses to be able to jump this height!

So – barbed wire for horses is absolutely out. Wire netting so often used for sheep is also useless and potentially dangerous for horses. In short, use your imagination and envisage whatever accident you can when examining premises for your horse's safety, whether fencing, stabling or general facilities where your horse is likely to go or be taken.

2.10 SHELTER

It always amazes me how little regard many horse owners and livery yard owners pay to providing shelter for their horses. Horses may be creatures of the open-air, but they definitely do need shelter facilities. Although, like any living body, they do acclimatize somewhat to being indoors or out, for good, humane management shelter really is needed from heat and sun in summer and wind, rain, snow and cold in winter.

It is often argued that a few trees here and there are sufficient shelter, but this is not the case. In summer, trees do not actually give much protection from the very significant discomfort created by insects unless they are in a thick belt or group of close-growing trees. Otherwise, the flies gather in the shade of the trees themselves and have a field-day irritating any horses who also happen to be there. Manes, forelocks and tails, in reality, offer poor protection against insects. Summer sheets can be used plus face shields or masks which improve the situation. In winter, insects are not the problem: wind and wet are. Here in the UK, our native ponies and cobs can tolerate our winter climate provided they are not clipped. Most other horses almost will certainly suffer, clipped or not, if exposed without adequate shelter to the average British winter – and, of course, there are countries that have much worse winters than we do.

The issue of winter rugs is fraught with problems. They need checking *at least* twice in every 24 hours and more often if the horse is out all the time. They must be an excellent fit for both size and shape, the back seam beginning in front of the withers and extending about a hand's width beyond the root of the tail. The seam must, of course, follow the curvature of the horse's back and the shaping must allow sideways fit for the shoulders and hips. Any signs of rubbing of the hair during checks are give-aways that the rug, albeit of the 'correct' size, does not fit that individual and, if not changed, could result in sore skin.

Remember that a horse in winter often wears his rug all the time except during exercise (and may have an exercise sheet then). This can certainly be quite stressful, resulting in discomfort, rubbing, frustration, soreness and pain – not what a caring owner wants for their horse. As well as the length already mentioned and the freedom of shoulders and hips, the fastenings on a rug are also important. Simply tightening them up may well keep the rug on and more or less in place but can also cause great discomfort to the horse. On the other hand, if they are too loose they can slip and hang in an uncomfortable position or even enable the horse to get a leg between a strap and his rug, or own body, which is dangerous.

As well as ensuring that his mane and coat hair lie smoothly under the rug, the straps securing the rug from front to back (and there are various designs) should allow the width of your hand between the strap and the rug, same for the leg straps or any fillet strap round the back of the thighs. At the front, the fastening can be adjusted comfortably freely if the rug is correctly shaped and fits well – that is that the horse can get his head down to eat off the floor or ground with only moderate pressure from the front fastening on his lower neck. Needless to say, one rug, particularly in wet weather, is not enough to ensure that he always has a dry rug to be changed into. (These remarks on fit also go for indoor clothing.)

2.11 SHELTER SHEDS

The best protection, and it will be well used I guarantee, is to provide your horses with a man-made shelter shed. If you buy a ready-made one, try to get a circular one which prevents a horse being cornered in the shed and attacked by another. Obviously, it is best to only leave out friends together, but arguments do happen.

The size of the shed for, say, two horses is a moot point. Anything is certainly better than nothing, but as a guide, from side to side the shed should be at least the size of a loose box and preferably 18 feet or about 5.5 metres wide but can be less from front to back. The open front should not take up all the front, so that horses can still get shelter if the wind changes direction. Basically, the shed should face south in winter and north in summer, but siting a shed with the front away from the prevailing wind is the over-riding requirement. There needs to be facilities inside for feeding hay or haylage although this can simply be placed on the ground. There are 'moveable' sheds available so that you can turn them round to face north in summer and south in winter, and I have seen one on skids that can be towed to a different area by a tractor if the entrance becomes poached.

If you can find an arrangement comprising, say, a barn opening on to a paddock or safely surfaced yard, this will be well-used by the horses. If you have your own premises you can perhaps create a facility with a shelter shed opening on to a surfaced, fenced area, in turn opening on to a paddock. The possibilities are endless and will be so much appreciated by the horses.

2.12 STABLES AND INDOOR ACCOMMODATION

Many horses spend much, even most, of their time inside their stable/ loose box so it is important that we make it as inviting and horse-friendly as possible. A few horses are still kept in stalls, that is tethered by the head at the back of the stall (which will be on average about 6 feet/2 metres wide although wider and narrower ones exist depending on the size of the horse. In stalls, the feed, hay and water points are all at the back of the stall so the horse can reach them easily when he wants to.

Square loose boxes, in which the horse can wander around freely, are the most usual way now of stabling horses. The British Horse Society recommends a measurement of 12 feet square for a horse, less for a pony. A larger box is needed for a stallion or a mare with foal at foot, also large foaling boxes. Many people would now regard 12 feet square as minimal and, within reason, the larger the box the better. An important fact often overlooked is the height of the box. The ceiling or roof needs to be high enough to prevent a rearing horse banging his head on it.

Ventilation in stables is very important because horses are naturally prone to respiratory irritations and diseases, so clean, fresh air, without draughts, is important. Badly managed bedding in any stabling can lead to the presence in the air of ammonia from the horses' urine, which has a very bad effect on the horses' eyes, respiratory tract and lungs, so careful attention to the bedding plus good ventilation and ample time outdoors for the horses is essential for their health. Leaving the double-leaved door with the top door open is insufficient in most cases and, to enable this night and day, mostly all year round, the stable should face away from the prevailing wind. There is usually a window on the same side of the door with a top opening flap which, again, should be open most of the time. This is the usual, most basic form of ventilation in basic standard loose boxes but can be improved on, for the health and interest of the horse.

Boxes with openings of various kinds on the sides and back walls allow the horse a variety of views and, of course, air flow, and can be adjusted according to the wind and rain direction. What most stabling is missing is roof ridge ventilation. If having stabling specially built or converted, try to have open-ridge type ventilation installed with a cowling on top to keep the rain out. This open ridge runs the whole length of the row of boxes with joining supports at various distances along the ridge. Because stale air rises, these provide excellent ventilation even without having the box windows open in bad weather. Individual ridge-roof ventilators can be fitted instead, if preferred, to each box. Stale, warm air rises and flows out of the space provided without causing draughts in the box below. When the horses are out, it is a good opportunity to open all ventilation points and really ventilate the horses' air space.

Bearing in mind the horse's natural need for company of his own kind, and the fact that he may spend many hours in his stable, it is good to house friendly horses in boxes with dividing walls low enough to allow them to touch maybe through vertical railings although not necessarily, but high enough to discourage them from trying to jump or scramble over them, depending on the height of the horse. There is nothing wrong with stabling two friendly horses or ponies in one large box so the horses can come in or go out as they wish and be in a fairly natural herd environment. Horses kept in groups in barns or any safe, large building, preferably leading on to a surfaced area or paddock, are living in an excellent environment for domestic working horses. Horses kept in domestic groups soon sort out their friends and this way of keeping them makes for, in my experience, settled, happy and sociable horses. The issue of relationships is always present, but sensible people – owners or staff – can arrange the groups so that only compatible ones are out in this way together. They can live this way indefinitely or just for a few enjoyable hours a day, maybe on a rota on a large yard, much to their advantage.

Group housing seems to be becoming more common and, provided the groups are selected wisely and the horses' basic needs are catered for, this is a better way of keeping most of them than isolated in individual boxes. The problems arise when newcomers or unfriendly horses are put out together: broken legs from kicks in these circumstances are far from unknown and almost always end in the victim being put down.

Overcrowding can also be a problem. As a youngster, I was taught that horses should only be turned loose in paddocks allowing half an acre per horse, which seems luxurious to the point of impossibility in modern conditions. The most important factor is certainly how well horses get on together. Newcomers should be turned out with one other calm and preferably socially senior horse first, then, if possible, maybe moved to an adjacent paddock to their intended one so the newcomer, in the presence of his 'mentor', can get to know the others over the fence, maybe bring one or two of them into the newcomer's paddock which should work owing to the presence of the other horse, and take it from there. Hacking out together is a traditional and effective way of introducing horses to each other, as well.

2.13 CONFINEMENT

There are times when a horse may need box rest for an injury or illness. If the horse is unwell enough, he will probably be glad of the privacy of his box, clean bedding, kind attention from humans, appropriate food and water and being made comfortable as regards temperature in his box, his rug being removed to rest his body, if the temperature permits this, gentle sponging of his face, sheath, under his/her tail and so on, but only light grooming should be done to avoid stressing him. Particular attention must be paid to picking out his feet as they will soon become packed with droppings if he is in most or all of the time. Skipping out also must be done several times a day, partly because of his feet but also his air quality.

It is always a help, if possible and appropriate, for him to have company of his favoured kind so that he does not feel isolated. Contentment as far as it can be provided can help recovery due to a calmer mind. If his box is big enough, a small pony friend can be in here with him. Cats are often sensitive to the well-being of horses who are off-colour and might perch on their doors, lie on their backs or just find a spot in the stable – or the manger – and it is obvious that the horses find this companionship very welcome.

2.14 GROUND CONDITIONS AND FOOTING

Horses left to themselves are pretty footsure and able to cope with most ground conditions. Naturally, of course, they roamed on soil and grassy areas which provided some 'give' and softened the impact of their hooves landing on the ground. They would also come across stoney areas, mud and rock-hard ground conditions in certain weather conditions. Many horses today dislike muddy conditions, to the point at which they will not approach, say, a water trough in a field because the area surrounding it has become poached and deeply muddy due to other horses approaching and leaving the trough in wet weather. The same applies to gateways. Mud can be pretty damaging to the skin on horses' lower legs and the thin skin on their bellies and between their hind legs if splashed up during faster paces. Cattle udder cream has been found by a friend of mine to be very effective at protecting horses' skin from mud in such conditions.

Ground conditions in general should be taken into account as regards basic management and during the horse's working times. Most of us know that fast work, even fast trotting, or in some cases any trotting, on hard surfaces like roads should be avoided because of the concussion to joints but also the danger of slipping. Deep going, usually mud but also soft, dry sand, are ground conditions that need to be avoided, if possible, otherwise a horse needs to be allowed largely to pick his own way and at walk only. Sharp stoney areas, as mentioned, should be avoided – even dismounting and leading is not proof against the horse injuring his feet.

Artificial surfaces are common now, of course, in outdoor manèges and indoor schools, and there are various different mixtures. The objective is to give the horse confidence with a secure footing – secure and not very deep but shock-absorbing and certainly non-slip and not inclined to pack in the feet. Schools indoor or out are convenient places to turn horses loose for a play and freedom when fields are too wet and two spells out per day are better than one, if possible. Many people do not like their schools being used for this purpose, but when there is no alternative it is the horses' well-being that matters more than the school surface which, admittedly at some expense, can always be topped up.

My first horse, whom I kept in the north Fylde on the coast of West Lancashire, soon grew used to carefully feeling his way, head down, through the smooth pebbles which lined the coastline on the way to the sand and sea, but, of course, no caring horse person would expect a horse to negotiate areas of sharp stones. Deep mud is anathema to most horses and, of course, areas where human-deposited litter may be buried.

2.15 NOISE LEVELS

In natural conditions, of course, horses do not experience any man-made sounds at all. They soon accustom themselves to them, such as traffic sounds (easily coming to recognise different people's car engines, for instance), aeroplanes, mowing machines, clipping machines, trains, sirens and so on. What I find is a generally misunderstood aspect of sound in horses' environments is that of radios playing in stable areas. It is understandable that we may well like the radio on when we are tending to the horses and yard work, but I have known many very sensitive and knowledgeable people in the past who have recognised that horses do not always like such sounds. During my time as a freelance writer, I was fortunate enough to be commissioned to visit some very highly regarded and famous stable yards in order to write about them and I frequently found that radios in many of them were restricted to half an hour at a time at a moderate volume. This was because it was found that after this length of time some of the horses started showing signs of stress such as head tossing, grinding teeth, box walking, stopping eating and so on.

One of my most enjoyable, educational and fascinating tasks was to follow the horses of racehorse trainer Gordon W. Richards some decades ago. I was at his yard every few weeks for a full year and he had the half-hour rule in operation morning and evening, and in the afternoons when the horses were resting and few humans were around, radios were not allowed at all. He told me that the music was mainly to keep the staff happy but many of the horses didn't like it, hence its being rationed.

It is not unusual to see competition horses, particularly show-jumpers, it seems, with cotton wool in their ears when competing to deaden the sounds of the crowds.

During the 1970s when Ireland's National Stud was led by veterinary surgeon and highly respected horseman Michael Osborne, I visited the stud several times and was particularly interested in the various scientific experiments they carried out there to better understand horse management, including behaviour and psychology. They had discovered that horses did not like any kind of pop music (or the human voice!) but loved gentle ballads and classical music, and, interestingly, military music. One stallion there at the time used to piaffe in his box to the latter.

I used to teach at a small yard very close to an airport and was interested to see that the horses there paid no attention at all to the deafening sound of aeroplanes flying overhead to land or take off. I was told that, at first, any newcomers to the yard would be initially not turned loose for a couple of days until they got used to the noise, then they would go out with the most 'immune' horses who paid no attention whatsoever to the din, and that the new ones would take their example from them and become plane-proof within a week or two.

Horses do have very acute hearing as part of their protection mechanism as prey animals, so making certain that they are not stressed by loud radios or music whenever possible, particularly if sustained and the horses cannot get away from it, such as when they are stabled, makes considerate horse sense.

2.16 RUGS, TACK AND OTHER EQUIPMENT

Most domestic horses have to wear some item of tack every day whether that is rugs or sheets, boots, saddles and cloths or pads, bridles, headcollars or halters. They have also to get used to other equipment from a young age, like buckets, grooming kit, brushes and forks, haynets and the general paraphernalia of stable and equestrian life.

The important factor in all this is to make sure that our equipment does its job but is also horse-friendly and is not a source of injury to horses. Leaving forks, brushes or, indeed, anything else in a horse's box, for instance, if we are called away for a short time is asking for trouble – and if there is any, horses will find it. At the time of writing, here in the UK there is a 'cost of living crisis' and probably in other countries, too. This has meant that various aspects of horse care and management have been cut down to save money. There is no doubt that horses now are very expensive to keep properly and some economies have to be made. It can be tricky deciding when enough is enough.

I have repeatedly found that one of the areas which is skimped is ensuring that a horse or pony's saddle fits him or her properly. At the start of lessons, I have many a time tactfully had to point out that a horse's saddle does not fit him properly and could be at best uncomfortable or, especially if worn for some time, probably painful, discussed calling in the local saddle fitter but have been told that the owner cannot afford it. Their answer to the problem, understandable enough but in many cases not appropriate, is to put various cloths and pads underneath which may relieve the pressure somewhat but can upset the balance of the saddle and so be a dubious solution to the problem. This is a difficult situation but, like veterinary and farriery services, should be regarded as unavoidable.

Other items of tack (there are qualified bridle fitters as well now) can be checked and possibly adjusted by owners or whoever is responsible for the horse's work and comfort. Today, bridles are excruciatingly tight and I really cannot understand why nothing seems to be done about it by 'the powers that be' – equestrian organisations of various sorts. In public competition, there are now moves afoot to encourage, or even enforce, kinder riding techniques, thankfully, but nothing seems to be done about a horse's tack which is so crucial to his comfort. Saddles are often put on too far forward, interfering with the movement of the top of the horse's shoulders and causing bruising there, also pulling the girth forward and causing pain and bruising behind the elbow from the girth as a result.

(The reason a saddle placed too far forward can bruise the tops of the horse's shoulders is because the shoulder blade swivels round when the attached foreleg moves. When, for instance, the left fore moves forward, the bottom of the shoulder bone/blade moves forward with the leg but the top of the shoulder blade moves backwards under the front of the saddle, and can be bruised by it. The shoulder blade needs to be free in this area, with the saddle placed correctly, so that, when the horse is standing still, the side of a hand can be fitted between the top of the shoulder blade and the front of the saddle. If the saddle is further forward than this, the pressure on the top of the shoulder blade will be certainly uncomfortable for the horse and maybe painful.)

The standard guidance of bridle fitting is usually ignored today. It states that we should be able to easily run a finger under all straps of the bridle, paying special attention to the browband, throatlatch and noseband, and allowing freedom around the base of the ears: in fact, we should be able to fit the sideways width of a hand between the throatlatch and the horse's round cheekbone. A snaffle bit or the bridoon (slim snaffle) of a double bridle should create no more than one wrinkle at the corners of a horse's mouth, a pelham should just touch them, and the curb bit of a double bridle should lie just low enough not to touch the corners of the mouth at all and lie under the bridoon in the mouth.

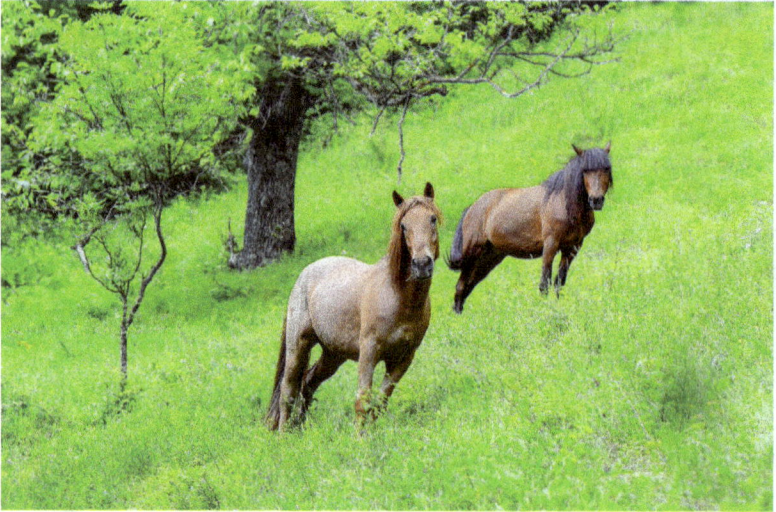

Figure 2.1 Any outdoor land used for giving horses some freedom needs at least one flat area. The strain of continually standing and moving on slopes stresses the horses' bodies and also does not provide them with a flat area on which to lie down to rest and sleep.

Source: (Shutterstock ID: 140452189)

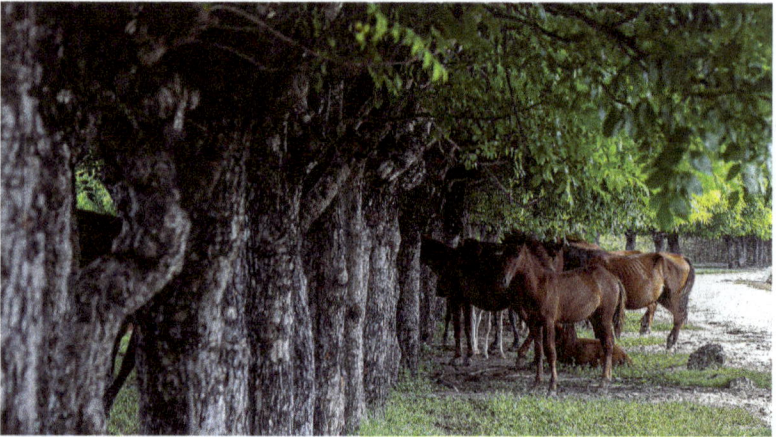

Figure 2.2 Shelter belts of trees are excellent for horses, although in certain, hot weather conditions they can become overcrowded with insects which torment the horses. Even a single, large tree with ample foliage is welcome in sunny weather. Horses need shelter from wind and rain, too, which a shelter belt on the windward side of a paddock can provide.

Source: (Shutterstock ID: 2450152235)

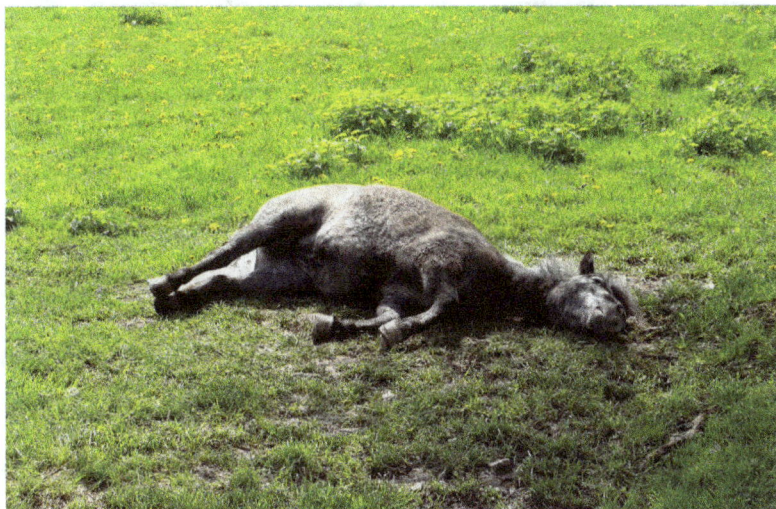

Figure 2.3 To actually sleep rather than just doze heavily, horses must lie flat out on the ground or stable floor. Stables must be large enough to permit this, and outdoor areas must provide ample, flat areas. Expert opinions vary as to how much actual sleep horses and ponies need per 24 hours, but generally four to seven hours is suggested.
Source: (Shutterstock ID: 53101330)

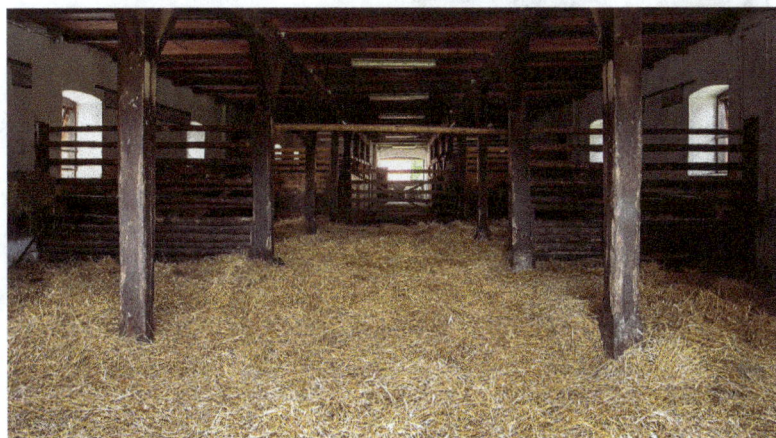

Figure 2.4 An excellent and welcome facility for horses' mental contentment and physical health is a facility like this, in which horses can be indoors or out, as they wish. The stables can be used to keep horses in, as required, or let them come and go if they wish to.
Source: (Shutterstock ID: 2005656191)

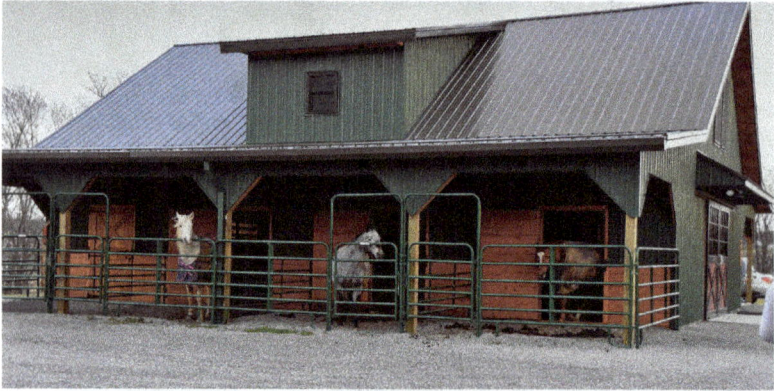

Figure 2.5 This type of arrangement can give the horses some freedom to come and go in and out of their boxes, when appropriate (e.g. with friendly horses), while restraining them when necessary.
Source: (Shutterstock ID: 2226713379)

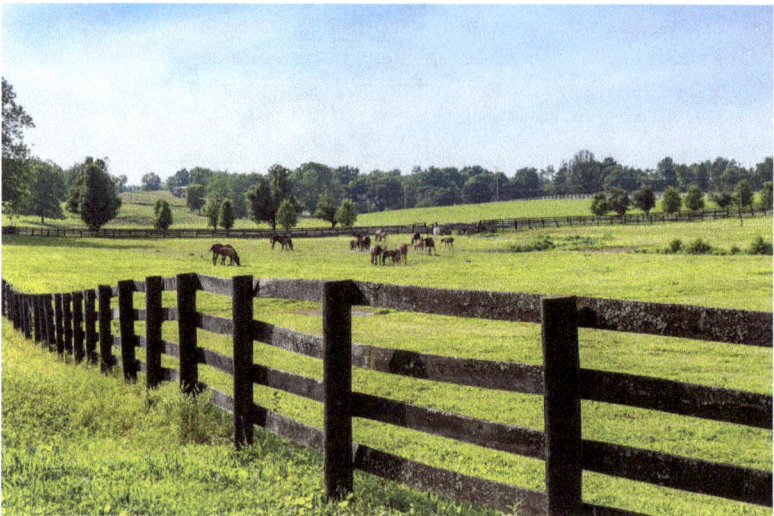

Figure 2.6 Although traditional post and rail fencing is still an excellent way of dividing grazing and exercise areas, the rails should always go on the *inside* of the posts. Horses often canter up and down fence boundaries and protruding posts can injure their shoulders and hips. Also, the top rail should always be level with the tops of the posts, so that, if horses try to jump out, they will not seriously injure their bellies on the protruding tops of the posts. As to height, fencing should be *at least* the height of the horses' withers to discourage them from jumping out, and usually considerably higher for stallions.
Source: (Shutterstock ID: 741091492)

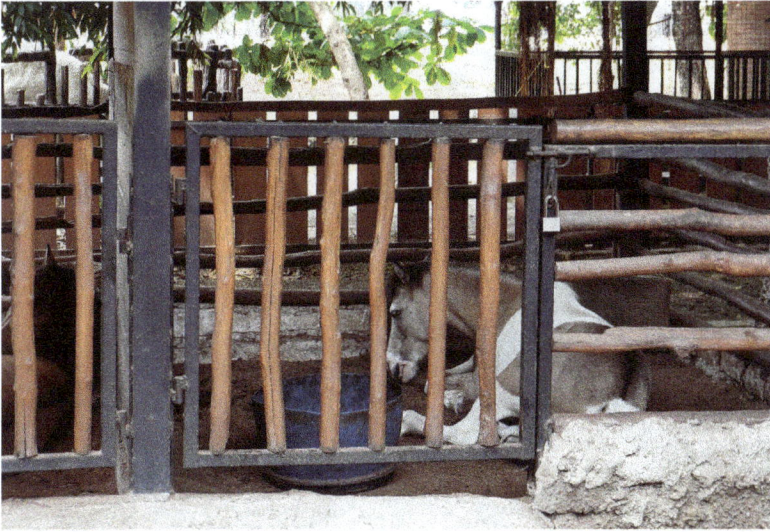

Figure 2.7 Horses used to being turned out in surfaced, fenced areas like this often feel sufficiently safe to lie down and sleep, and they are a useful alternative to grassland when the land is too wet to turn out.

Source: (Shutterstock ID: 2499440177)

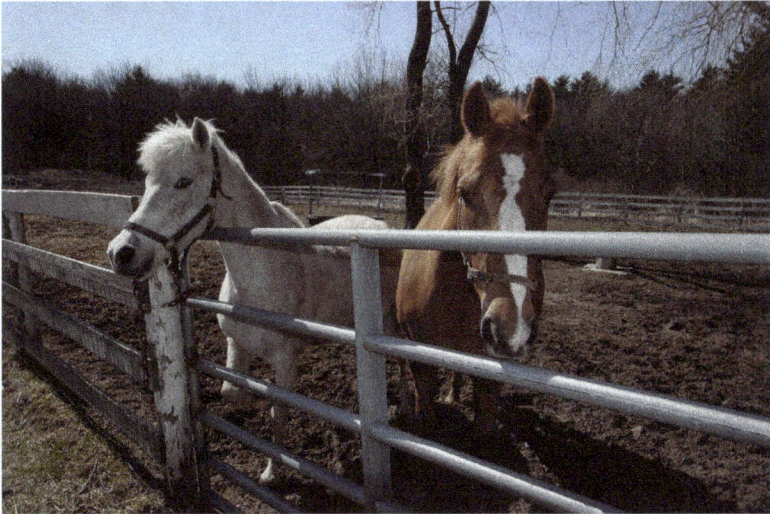

Figure 2.8 Although many people do not like turning horses out on to their manèges or schools for fear of too much damage to the expensive surface, the horses' well-being should come first, and any suitable area used when grass turnout is unavailable.

Source: (Shutterstock ID: 3008288)

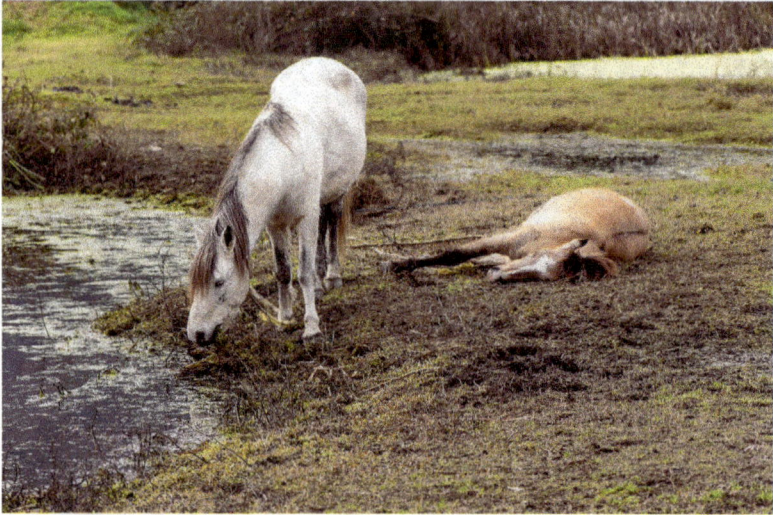

Figure 2.9 It is understandable that owners will want their horses in safe areas as far as possible. However, horses are not stupid and areas some might see as potentially dangerous often offer interesting and varied surroundings for horses.

Source: (Shutterstock ID: 2419006407)

Ill-fitting rugs and sheets that not only do not fit the horse but do not stay in position during wear cause a great deal of discomfort to a horse, who is usually wearing them for several hours, if not all the time, whether in or out. And yes, there *are* trained rug-fitters too, now, who can help you ensure your horse's protection and comfort, usually employed by quality tack shops.

I am sure most people do not realise the discomfort, even pain, that ill-fitting or unsuitable tack and rugs cause to a horse, even by just putting them on and adjusting them wrongly, and I hope that more people will seek out the services of the right help to ensure that their horses are comfortable, happy, able to enjoy their lives at work, rest and play, and perform for us in comfort.

2.17 SAFE ENVIRONMENT

It is amazing how easily horses and particularly, it seems, ponies find trouble. It really can save you time, money and lost riding time if you take a few minutes and make it a habit to see that your horses' environments are safe and unlikely to cause them injury. Everything from protruding

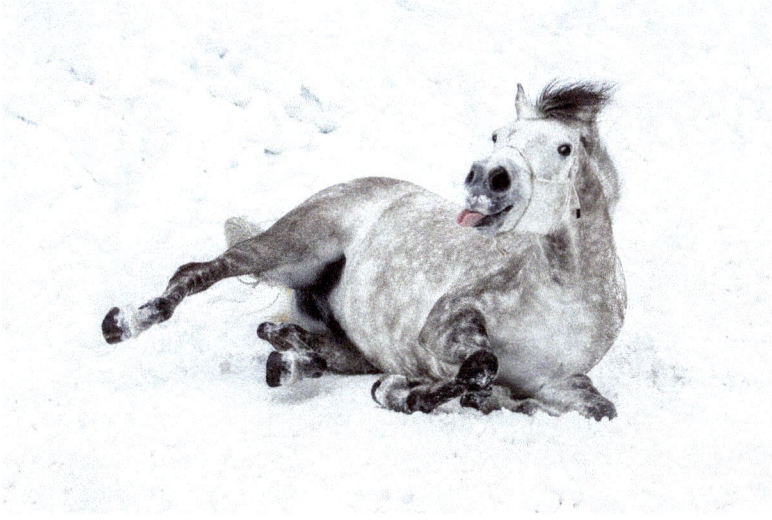

Figure 2.10 Most horses love playing and rolling in snow, especially in regions that don't see much of it. It is a good idea to generously oil the underside of the horses' hooves before turning them out because snow can pack firmly in the feet and prevent the horses moving around freely (or at all) to keep warm.

Source: (Shutterstock ID: 1497550094)

nails to poisonous plants needs to be spotted and sorted out to avoid injury and expensive vet's bills. Polythene bags wafting about the yard, general litter, equipment left in fields, buckets, headcollars, ropes and grooming kits left lying around, in fact just about anything you can think of can cause injury to a horse either directly or by his falling or stumbling over it.

More major things like doors left open protruding into the yard, the feed room door left open if there is a horse wandering freely in the yard, wheelbarrows standing around, brushes or forks left lying on the ground can all cause accidents and injuries. Other things are broken fencing, which can injure the horse himself and allow escape from a field to who knows where. Carelessly leaving a stable door open can, and has, led to the death of a horse and the injury of a person on a public road.

Making safety a state of mind, particularly when carelessness is involved, can save lives.

Health

Three

It is clear to all of us that without reasonable to good health none of us, animal or human, can do very much in life. There is a lot to be said for encompassing more of nature into our lives and, here, we must admit that most people keep horses in very or fairly unnatural conditions. To horses' advantages, they are intelligent and adaptable animals, albeit with brains that are not structured, and therefore do not work entirely like ours (see Part 4).

Horses evolved to live out in the open mainly, using shelter facilities when needed and if available. There are, strictly speaking, no wild horses left on earth, those roaming and living a free life being technically termed 'feral', even the Przewalski horses, meaning that at some point in their history Man has interfered with their lives, perhaps to the extent of domesticating them and producing animals that are more tolerant of humans than wild ones. Wild animals and their ancestors have never been domesticated but all horses and ponies, even if living wild now, have at some point been domesticated or stem from previously domesticated ancestors. Their characteristics and behaviour seem identical to truly wild horses, according to historical descriptions from hundreds, even thousands, of years ago and modern domestic horses soon revert to their ancestors' behaviour and lifestyle when the opportunity arises.

3.1 BACK TO 'NATURE'

Many years ago, in my early 20s, I had at last succeeded in buying my own horse and kept him on livery at the home of a friend-of-a-friend. There were grass turnout facilities there, of course, but they could not be described as anywhere near natural conditions – just fenced grass paddocks so ubiquitous everywhere. A local farmer offered us the use of about 30 acres on which to turn out our eight horses for the summer. There were lots of close-growing trees for shelter, two troughs of piped water, and hedges and wooden post and rails instead of wire fencing. Most importantly, the land had not been seeded with sugar-rich ryegrass

DOI: 10.1201/9781003396376-4

but was the much more natural meadow grass, with different types of grasses so welcomed by horses. Naturally, we jumped at the chance of giving our horses this opportunity of a 'natural' summer life, even though the land was rather too far from their stables to bring them in and out if we wanted to ride. We chose not to ride, of course, but to leave them out at night and give the horses, some of them point-to-pointers, the chance of a well-earned rest, out 24 hours a day doing what comes naturally.

The horses' eyes popped out on stalks when they were taken through the main gate and saw their new home. They wasted no time in cantering off to the horizon to investigate the surroundings and facilities. We hung around for half an hour watching them investigating everywhere, then left them to enjoy their first night out. Next morning, two of us went to see how they had fared and found them in a loose herd three fields away. When they recognised us, our two horses came to greet us as usual but the others, knowing we weren't 'their' people, saw we were there but carried on grazing. All was well, the troughs were working properly and so we left. Someone checked on the horses once or twice every day and I did not see my horse for two days after their turnout. He looked at me, seemed to hesitate for a few seconds, then came to me as usual (he knew that I never carry titbits).

We found it really interesting to note their gradual change in behaviour over the weeks. They formed two herds and, although they mixed about a bit, basically they kept to a group of five and one of three, mixed mares and geldings. Both groups had one older horse in it, presumably for leadership and protection. My youngish horse was in the group of five, with one older mare leading it. We noticed that, close though we felt we were with our horses, the horses took longer and longer to come over and see us when we visited until, one day, they didn't come over at all, despite seeing our approach. They did welcome us, all being in one larger group, when we reached them, nuzzled us but not, apparently, for treats and carried on socialising and grazing.

This became the norm, until, one day, they actually moved away when we arrived (different people attended every day). The two people concerned did not try to stop them (what use would that have been?!) but diverted away and ahead, going round the top of the group several yards away and not looking at them. One horse came over but not the lead horse, stayed for a few minutes, then returned to the herd. Over the weeks, the horses fell into a semi-feral attitude and way of life. They did not make concerted efforts to move away when we arrived but were not

61 Health

particularly interested in our arrival. I was pretty hurt when, one day, my horse hardly paid me any attention at all! The feeling emanating from the horses was one of peaceful, confident, established independence. After all, they did have everything they wanted – grass and trees to browse, shelter, water, ample space (all the interior gates being left open), relative safety (the gate to the road being padlocked and the horses being out of sight of the general public) and plenty of land to roam over.

Although they did not show us any aggression or move away, as some might when being caught in the home paddocks for work, they just accepted we were visiting and they were staying. We noticed that they seemed to develop a 'herd appearance' of being let down, sassy but not, thank goodness, fat, sleek summer coats and not particularly dirty from grease or material such as soil picked up when rolling. Their manes and tails grew, as did their feet but, interestingly, the farrier only needed to come and trim (no shoes, of course) once during their 16 weeks out. There were hard paths on some parts of their holiday home which they used regularly so this helped keep the horn down.

I had been concerned about there being no man-made shelter on the fields and the horses being badly irritated by insects but, strangely, this did not seem to be happening. The main tree cover was pretty dense and was, in fact, a small wood. Flies are usually attracted under trees and, so, to any animals shading themselves there from summer sun, but our horses did not seem much bothered by them at all. The woodland was mixed and the horses browsed the leaves readily, there being little grass on the wood's floor.

Their holiday diet of just meadow grass and water, plus presumably the space, company, freedom and leisure to suit themselves, was all perfect for equines. This is the kind of life they were meant to lead with the notable exception of being preyed upon. From the road, the horses could not be seen on their allotted land so we weren't worried about out-of-control dogs harassing them, or of their being stolen (although I have to say I would not be so nonchalant today). Nutritionally, meadow grass, with its lower nutrient and especially sugar level than ryegrass and its wide variety of grasses and other tasty plants such as dandelions and others, suited our horses perfectly, and their appearance and aura, described earlier, showed that they had greatly benefited from the break and their surroundings and, particularly, their ability to graze the right sort of grass, to forage at will for many hours a day which is their birthright.

Horses handle boredom badly and eating is certainly the activity they evolved to do most of, for their minds and not only their appetites and bodies. They only sleep for roughly six hours a night and both want and need occupation. Heads down grazing and with eyes high up towards the sides of their heads means they can see almost all around themselves, their narrow legs not offering much obstruction to the view of predators approaching so they can stoke up their nutrient needs and keep watch at the same time.

On the day, at the end of September, when they were to come back to the stable yard, we all turned up with headcollars and ropes to bring them back to the stable yard and, strangely, there wasn't one single objection. They all stood for their headcollars and, when all were ready, they led calmly down to the road gate for the half-hour walk to the yard. On being returned to their usual (spruced up) stables, there was a little suspicion at the different smell due to wood treatments, cleaning materials and so on, but no one refused to enter their box, where deep beds, hay and water were waiting. Strangely again, after just a little whinnying to each other, they settled to eat the hay. This was lunchtime, and, after an hour, they were all turned out variously in the paddocks to maintain grass for their digestive health, but in the friendship pairings that had become apparent during the summer. The horses all slotted back into yard routine after a day or so, which we weren't sure would happen, but it did. They remembered not only where they were but also the timings of the different yard activities and their associated noises such as buckets rattling at feeding times.

What did we humans learn from this long summer holiday for our horses?

1. The first thing was how quickly, a matter of days really, these clearly domesticated horses, who were used to being turned out but spent rather more time in stables than paddocks, reverted to feral herd behaviour and mindset, and relied on their own company rather than looking to humans for their needs.
2. The second thing was how clearly the break had benefited them and how they all developed the same 'look' about them – let down, roughish, shining with health and happiness, confident and sort of 'established' – a safe, self-contained herd of mares and geldings, or rather two associating smaller ones of their own choosing.
3. The third thing was how there were no objections at all, or even apparent disappointment, when they were brought back to the stable

yard months later, just as the weather began to change (perhaps that had something to do with their willing attitude towards coming in!) and just settled in their familiar boxes to eat their hay – nothing too rich to start with; we managed to get some good meadow hay from the farmer who rented us the land. Those horses going on to hard work during the winter eventually would be gradually changed over to seed hay.

I think a good deal of the horses' calm behaviour when coming home again was due to the fact that they knew us all (and quickly got the hang of their summer landscape) and associated us and the stable yard, when they returned, with security, food, everyone present who should be and, simply, back to the old lifestyle – not to mention protection from the upcoming winter weather which they doubtless sensed was coming.

3.2 THE 'INNER HORSE'

The old remedy for horses with some health problems – 'Dr Green' – meant that time out in the field, particularly during spring, summer and autumn (depending on where in the world we are) was if not the only medicine needed at least a major advantage in improving a horse's well-being and, through a happier and calmer mind plus the pleasure of eating natural food and the actions of grazing, Dr Green could and, of course, still can form a most important boost to a horse's mind and body. Freedom, most likely with friendly horses for company as in nature and with access to grazing and perhaps browsing, is a sure fire way, with most equines, to settle the mind, relax the body and lift the spirits. (All these states of being also are beneficial to the physical health of any creature, including humans.) Dr Green was and still is so often right.

Of course, horses, particularly domestic ones used to stabling, do seek shelter from significantly adverse weather conditions – burning hot sun, freezing cold, wind, rain and snow are all significant challenges for them as for us. Exposure to any bad living conditions whether that is the climate and weather, over-confinement, too much food, too little food, inappropriate food, stressful work of whatever kind, fear of humans or other horses or animals can all physically and mentally bring down a horse's welfare and well-being levels, as they can with any other creature, including humans. There is a lot more to looking after horses than feeding, grooming, exercising, mucking out and having visits from the vet, farrier and any other therapist.

The healthiest horses are often the happiest because misery, anxiety, sadness, fear and any other negative emotion can certainly bring with it poorer physical health in humans and animals. This part of the book is a guide to recognising good and poor health in horses, both physical and mental, so that you will know when to seek expert advice, most commonly from your veterinary surgeon/veterinarian.

3.3 DEVELOPING YOUR SIXTH SENSE

How does your horse seem at first glance when you haven't seen him for a while? Do you ask yourself how he seems or just assume he is alright until something obvious makes itself known?

If your relationship with your horse is a close one, you will know as soon as you see him how he is feeling at that moment, not just what mood or state of mind he is in but whether he is quite well, a bit off-colour or undeniably sick. If your relationship is not that close or if you have not been together long, you may not know or feel immediately how the horse is but if you 'open your mind', as it were, not assuming he is alright, and just assess him objectively, you will gradually come to know him in his different states and confidently ask for help when he is below par. Sometimes you can see when something is not right. At other times you may just get a feeling, so then, by keeping an eye on him, his condition will gradually become clearer to you.

Most of us are so busy today that we never think, or think we have the time, to stop and stare, as it were. Life seems to get busier and busier, and often we are so pre-occupied with what we have to do during the rest of that day that we think that we don't have the time to live and be in the moment. But doing this is so valuable, particularly when we want to develop that almost spiritual or intuitive Sixth Sense that so often comes to our rescue – if we let it.

People who have allowed that sense to develop in them can know almost immediately, even with horses they have never met before, what state of mental or physical health they are in, not necessarily what exactly is wrong with them if anything, but just a certainty that something is not right. When a horse is our own, or one we know well, perhaps belonging to a friend, we can know as soon as we set eyes on him or her that something is amiss. Conversely, just a glance can tell us at once that all is right with his world. It may be a matter of actual mental or physical health, or just what mood he is in, but if we get 'that feeling' we can bet that most of the time it is correct, for better or worse. The important thing is not to guide it, but to keep an open mind and just let it swim around and guide you. The more you let it help you, without imagining anything to influence it, the better you will be able to rely on it and take things from there.

3.4 RECOGNISING GOOD AND POOR HEALTH AND CONDITION

Horses, as we know, naturally are prey animals. As such their inborn inclination is to try to hide injuries, lameness, sickness, in fact any weaknesses that a hunting predator looking to feed its family could spot as making a horse easy to overcome. In domestic conditions, it may be that they are more inclined to let their natural state of being show but many do tend to fight on and continue to keep up with their friends in the field, or to work for us, if they possibly can. Some changes of behaviour are obvious such as, whether in or out, is your horse lying down more than usual and looking unwell rather than sleepy, or is he standing up but with his head low and eyes half closed? Both these can mean a horse is not feeling his normal, healthy self, particularly if the horse shows no interest when someone approaches him.

Therefore, it is really important that we make regular observations of our horses, note every little change and do a fairly comprehensive health check every week. This does not mean an expensive vet visit and check-up every time: you can easily do it yourself, and keep a record of what you find in a special book for the purpose, or digitally on computer or whatever device you use.

3.5 SIGNS OF GOOD AND POOR HEALTH

A happy, healthy horse will be interested in his surroundings and what is going on round about. His eyes will be bright and his ears usually pointed to whatever he is paying attention to. There will be no abnormal discharge from his nostrils: a normal discharge is simply a slight, watery trickle. Even if you think he is dirty from rolling while out, his coat should be nevertheless basically fairly bright and, according to the time of year, smooth and flat in warm weather or thicker and cushioning if in its longer winter form. A 'staring' coat, that is, one that feels rough, not particularly pliable, and with the hairs seeming to be standing out from the skin somewhat, is indicative of poor condition and health. When he moves, he should do so confidently with an even beat depending on which gait he is in. Very often, owners complain that their horse is 'lazy today' when actually his feet are hurting him and he could be found to be starting with laminitis, or his feet could need trimming and/or shoeing.

Skin conditions plague horses just as they can any other animal. Badly fitting clothing is a prime cause of not only maddening itching or rubbing but of soreness. The coat hair does not protect the skin from the artificial pressure and rubbing of clothing that does not fit or has moved around and, due to lack of attention, has not been corrected. If the horse is rubbing or biting himself, with or without clothing, there is probably a skin complaint that needs looking into. These can be transferred from another horse, be due to a sensitivity to, say, shampoo or other coat dressings, or be part of the symptoms of a disease. Whatever, he needs veterinary attention to determine the cause and procure appropriate treatment.

Your horse should move around his box or paddock freely and easily. When standing, his forefeet should be firmly planted evenly together: he may rest one hind leg alternately. If he is constantly shifting his stance as though trying to get comfortable, there could well be a problem. Obviously, if his gait is uneven, if he is very slightly lame or clearly so, this needs attention. Any swelling on the legs can indicate trouble. Also, feel with the backs of your fingers all round each hoof to see if you can detect any abnormal heat in the foot: this can indicate laminitis which often occurs in pairs of feet, front or rear, and can come on very quickly.

If your horse is leaving feed and hay and usually cleans up, there will almost certainly be a problem with your horse or with the feed. Horses have delicate digestive systems (and respiratory systems) and often wisely refuse poor quality and particularly mouldy, dusty or sour feed or hay. Hay is often stored in open barns but must be kept dry and well ventilated. An open-fronted barn should face away from the prevailing wind and weather for this reason. 'Short' or manger feed such as grain or commercially prepared feed is commonly kept in a special feed room in bins with sound lids, all usually metal to prevent rats gnawing through the bin to get at the feed. Rinse them out well, and let them dry before refilling with fresh feed.

A basic but good weekly check is given below. Really, you need a friend to lead your horse around, trot him up, stand him and so on while you assess how he is. If your friend is more experienced and knowledgeable than you are, I am sure that, in the interests of both you and your horse, he or she would be pleased if you did the handling and they did the assessing.

Choose an area with a level, hard and smooth surface for standing and trotting up, ideally out of the weather if it is bad because even this type of discomfort can affect and change a horse's way of going, as can feet

67 Health

in need of shoeing or trimming. Hard, smooth going is ideal for picking up even slight lameness, which is more likely to show up on a circle or bend than a straight line, if such is possible. Even very slight lameness in trot shows up on a bend. Your horse should wear a bridle and bit, or a well-fitting halter or headcollar and, if the weather is poor, can wear a rug. I suggest you proceed as follows.

If you haven't done so already, go into your horse's stable, or bring him in from the field if he is out, and use that Sixth Sense to assess how you think he is feeling. If a horse outdoors has been standing or lying in one place for a long time, say over half an hour, suspect that something is wrong. If a stabled horse is standing at the back of his box looking uninterested, or has been lying down particularly during the day for that length of time, again there could be a problem. It is always best to be on the safe side and check. Obviously, if a recumbent horse has trouble getting up there is probably a problem, usually in his legs or hip and shoulder joints.

Ask yourself: Is he interested in you – or your pockets?! If he is sleepy or resting, does he perk up when you appear? Is he interested in his surroundings? Does he have a calm facial expression, does he seem sleepy or, more suspect, dull and not interested in his surroundings? Conversely, does he look worried or frightened with wide eyes? Is he tossing his head and ill at ease? Are his ears mobile and moving around towards what he is interested in, or are they held loosely, sideways, meaning he doesn't feel well, or held back with a strained facial expression, which can mean he is in pain. If you spot him grinding his teeth, this usually indicates fairly high pain levels as can moaning, snorting or uneven breathing.

A horse's tail is also informative: if it is clamped between his buttocks, thrashing or held out stiffly, this is a sure sign he feels unwell or is in pain. If he is moving from foot to foot, this clearly indicates hoof pain and if he is snatching at his sides, getting up and down and/or frequently rolling, he has quite severe abdominal pain.

(If ever your horse seems alright and you get him ready to ride but, on mounting and setting off, find him sluggish or in any way not moving like his usual self, dismount and perform some checks, ideally with an experienced person if you yourself are, perhaps, not very experienced, or simply to get a valuable second opinion.)

All these signs and, in fact, anything abnormal about him, which you will probably spot within seconds or a very few minutes of seeing him, can indicate trouble and mean a call to the vet, with a probable visit.

Whether your horse is in or out, remove any clothing he is wearing and check his physical body condition – that is, how well covered he is by fat. Today, overweight seems to be more common than underweight and can cause more health issues. A quick and easy guide to good, average weight or body condition, as we call it, for any horse or pony is that you should be able to feel his ribs fairly easily but not see them, unless he is turning away from you.

So, if you can see his ribs when he is just standing, or moving in a straight line, he is probably underweight, but if you cannot feel his ribs easily but have to press around, he is probably too fat.

There is a view that very fit horses often show their ribs and this is correct for them, but I have veterinary assurance that this is most unlikely. A horse can and should be well covered and muscled up for work but not be thin. Conversely, there are still too many fat animals presented in the show ring, and in life in general. Fortunately, at the time of writing, there is increasing publicity about the dangers of obesity: some shows have made rulings about animals' condition as well as riders who are too heavy for their mounts. Unfortunately, behind the scenes (outside the warming up area) there are still problems with too-heavy adults warming up children's ponies, which is harmful for the ponies, selfish and dishonest.

Three basic and informative health indicators to check are your horse's temperature, pulse and respiration rates, his TPR rates as they are known.

Taking your horse's temperature weekly or whenever you suspect he is off-colour is a valuable guide to his health. There are various types of thermometers, from the traditional mercury one to modern electronic ones with display screens. Obviously, follow the instructions for use of whatever type of thermometer you buy.

The older-type mercury thermometer is currently the cheapest, still widely used and very accurate. Simply remove it from its case *not* by holding the bulb, shake the mercury well down, lubricate the bulb and a little way above it with Vaseline or by spitting on it. Stand by the horse's tail, pulling the dock *towards* you. Carefully insert the thermometer horizontally by means of a back-and-forth twirling movement, pushing it into the anus at the same time, smoothly until it is about halfway in. Do not let go! Keep it in place for a *minimum* of one minute and preferably two or three minutes. Smoothly withdraw it and read off the horse's temperature which, to be normal, should be 99 to 101.5 degrees Fahrenheit or 37.2 to 38.6 degrees Centigrade. If the temperature is a degree or more above or below these figures, it would be advisable to ring your vet for advice: he or she probably will want to know about other symptoms the horse may be showing.

Your horse's pulse is, obviously, a way of checking on his heart rate – its nature, such as if it is pounding or weak, and whether it is faster or slower than normal. Taking your horse's pulse is not difficult and is a valuable check on his health. It only takes a short while. The most common place at which to count the beats or pulses of the blood passing through a main artery is on the lower edge of the bottom jawbone close to the rounded cheekbone. Put the tips of your four fingers of one hand together and feel along the bone for the pulses. As the rate for a healthy, mature horse is 35 to 45 beats per minute, you need to keep your fingers in place for two or three seconds to see if you have found the right spot. Pass your free arm under his throat and steady his head with your hand on the front of his face as you feel around with the fingertips of your other hand.

The normal rate may be slightly slower in older horses and faster in youngsters and ponies. It is affected by physical condition, exercise and work, the outside temperature, whether the horse is excited or calm, and by disease.

To check your horse's respiration rate, stand behind him a little way back and to one side so that, if you are standing on the left, you can see his right side rising and falling as he breathes. This is best done in the stable, or somewhere quiet when he is relaxed. The normal rate of each in-out breath (counted as one breath) is 8 to 12 breaths per minute for a mature horse, maybe slower for older ones and faster for youngsters and ponies. Obviously, do not take his respiration rate straight after work but when he is rested, calm and not excited.

Injuries can vary from strains and sprains, cuts and tears of the skin, lumps and bumps, sprained tendons or ligaments or any other 'invasions' of his body. As advised earlier, one of your most helpful and valuable companions is a good, up-to-date veterinary book which can give you much valuable advice, not just dealing with cuts and bruises or deciding whether or not your horse is lame. Obviously, injuries should be treated appropriately as soon as they are spotted during your daily and weekly checks. You will get into the habit of quickly looking for and dealing with them during your daily care of your horse. Don't neglect them because infection can soon set into even a seemingly insignificant injury. Check with an experienced person or ring your veterinary practice, depending on how major or minor the injury is.

First aid for any condition will probably be covered in your veterinary book. Appropriate, prompt first aid can go a long way to setting your horse on the road to recovery before any further veterinary treatment, and it is well worthwhile becoming adept at this. Keep a first aid book at the stable yard if you keep your horse at livery so that it is quickly available when needed, together with whatever equipment it recommends you have to hand, such as buckets, salt, antiseptics, bathing equipment, your thermometer and so on, and keep your supplies stocked up. You can buy fully stocked first aid kits online or from any good tack shop and could bless the day you bought one.

First aid may be all that is needed for slight problems but, when conditions demand such as with cuts or tears that go deeper than the second layer of skin or bleed a good deal, obvious lameness or a horse clearly feeling unwell, do not delay in calling the vet. Yes, veterinary care is very expensive today, but it is probably the most important aspect of your horse's care to budget for and, along with annual vaccinations, worming and so on, should not be regarded as an extra.

The issue of veterinary insurance is a real bugbear these days. Insurance companies' rates have risen alarmingly in recent years, and companies are getting more and more selective about excluding various conditions from their policies once a horse has suffered from them. Even an old scar on a leg from an accident, rather than an illness, can cause a company to try to exclude any disorder of any of the horse's four legs, for instance. I have more than once found veterinary surgeons to be most helpful in reversing an insurance company's opinion on this and similar issues, so it is worth asking your vet's advice and by no means accepting the first premium quote you are given.

Years ago, I had a vet whose 'hobby horse' was unreasonable insurance quotes and he saved me a considerable sum of money on the insurance for a new horse with a scar on one leg. The previous owner told me it had been a minor cut, but the insurance company jumped on the chance to exclude all four legs from any injury at all! My vet rang them up (out of my hearing!), and I was subsequently given a much lower quote. People have various ways of ensuring the money is available for insurance premiums. Some do not report minor cases as it is cheaper to pay the vet for, say, one or two visits. Others do not insure their horses at all but pay what would be the monthly premium into a separate bank account which builds up over time, of course, and may well cover a horse's veterinary needs unless a very serious condition occurs. The latter situation is quite rare, so they feel it worthwhile taking that gamble.

Mental and psychological issues are dealt with in Parts 4 and 5. Here, we can just say that any abnormal behaviour for your individual horse can signal some problem or other. Stereotypical behaviour, formerly called 'stable vices', are not the fault of the horse and he should not be punished for performing them, as I have seen done. It is now widely believed that it is best to allow the horse to perform them as a release and to change his way of living to try to find some method that will ease his mind and reduce his stereotypies. It is often the case that, even in what has been called 'brain damaged' horses very prone to various behaviours, coming up with a happy and rewarding lifestyle for them can often greatly reduce the performance of stereotypies. It is also a fallacy that 'vices are catching'. If several horses in one yard are performing stereotypies it is probably the management that is seriously at fault.

However, many years ago I visited a rescue centre for horses, many of whom performed stereotypies whenever they were stabled, even for a relatively short time. This kind of situation is impossible to eradicate but, with good management that makes horses happy and settled, stereotypies can certainly be reduced. It is actually *bad* management to prevent an affected horse performing his 'vice' and can certainly make him worse: the answer is always to keep him or her happy, settled, free from worry, fear, hunger, loneliness and so on. Such horses, when stabled in individual loose boxes, often feel isolated. As such, they should never be stabled next to a horse they dislike or are frightened of but, quite the opposite, it is best to stable them next to a friend, and ideally so that they are able to touch and sniff each other, perhaps through railings on the upper half of the dividing wall instead of having a solid wall. Stable manufacturers, as shown by their advertisements in the equestrian press, seem to be very slow to amend their designs to allow for normal equine interactions but most stables can be adapted to allow horses adequate round-the-clock contact with friendly neighbours, and the horses will be happier and healthier for that.

As a matter of interest, many years ago I qualified as an equine shiatsu practitioner and used to visit a local equine rescue sanctuary that had many horses with behavioural issues due to bad management in the past. One mare I treated (an ex-racehorse) never stopped box walking when stabled but, after just one treatment, one of the grooms told me that, for an hour after my first visit, she stopped tramping around her box and stood with her head down, dozing peacefully, something the groom had never seen her do before. Shiatsu has the same benefits as acupuncture

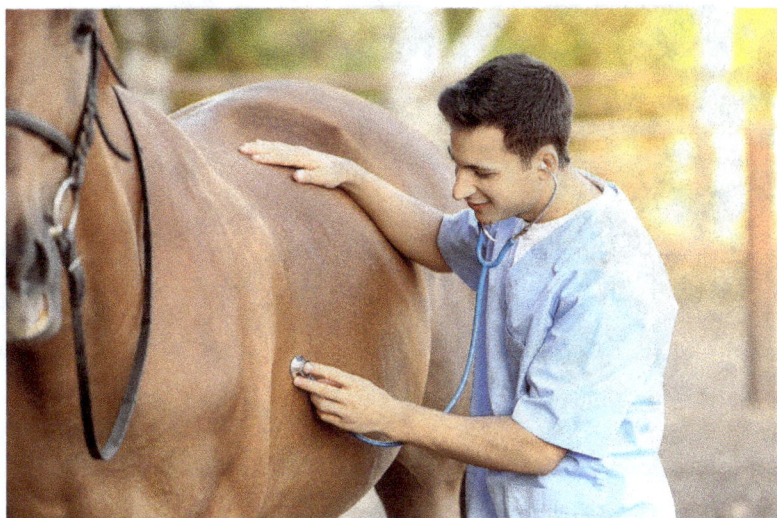

Figure 3.1 Veterinary services are expensive for many owners today, but frequent veterinary attention is essential for some horses. Most responsible yard owners arrange for regular vet visits to check on the horses, on vet's advice but possibly once every three to six months. Any good veterinary book will give readers details of how to do a more frequent health check themselves, or a vet would explain what is needed.
Source: (Shutterstock ID: 2083400317)

but without the needles. We use massage and pressure points using just our hands, and it has very noticeable corrective and calming, reassuring effects on horses with stereotypies and other behavioural problems. The society's website where you can find much information and the nearest practitioner to you is www.equineshiatsu.org.

Handling sick, suffering and injured horses can be very difficult and upsetting, even frightening, for many owners. Any good veterinary or first aid book should give advice on handling stressed and frightened horses, and you may well need to call in other genuinely competent help, such as your veterinary practice's staff. Veterinary surgeons these days are very ready to administer sedatives, where appropriate, to handle such horses, rather than restraining them by various physical means. This is a safety issue and enables them to treat horses without objection from the horse, or creating adverse associations. A struggling horse can make matters worse and old methods of physical restraint can hurt and frighten them, making them permanently difficult to handle even when well. It is worth

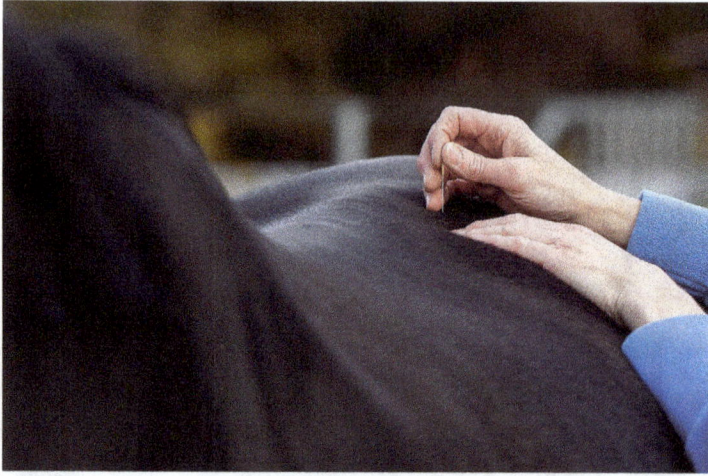

Figure 3.2 Acupuncture, shown being carried out here, is regarded as a complementary therapy but is sometimes used, and/or recommended, by conventional veterinary practitioners as well. It is related to acupressure and shiatsu and works on pressure points and meridians ('lines') of energy flow to promote good health and well-being. Many people are sceptical of such therapies but, in the author's long experience, they can help considerably.
Source: (Shutterstock ID: 1694092183)

researching up in your books and online how to deal with this issue, but, as so often, your vet is an excellent source of advice. Many vets when treating horses usually try milder methods of physical restraint but, wisely, will not get into a situation in which a horse is becoming really difficult to handle (and we can't blame the horse). In such cases, the vet will probably administer a sedative for safety and effectiveness of treatment.

When giving your horse prescribed care in the absence of your vet, follow his or her prior advice and try to get the help of another experienced horse owner. Confident, caring persistence often calms horses and allows you to do your part in helping them.

Diagnosis methods, treatment protocols and prognosis are certainly the field of your vet. We can learn so much by listening to our vet, asking questions about these very specialised processes and learning ourselves more about horses and maintaining their well-being. Veterinary science research is constantly ongoing, and new methods and ideas become available all the time. Although we can 'diagnose' lameness in a horse and decide what to

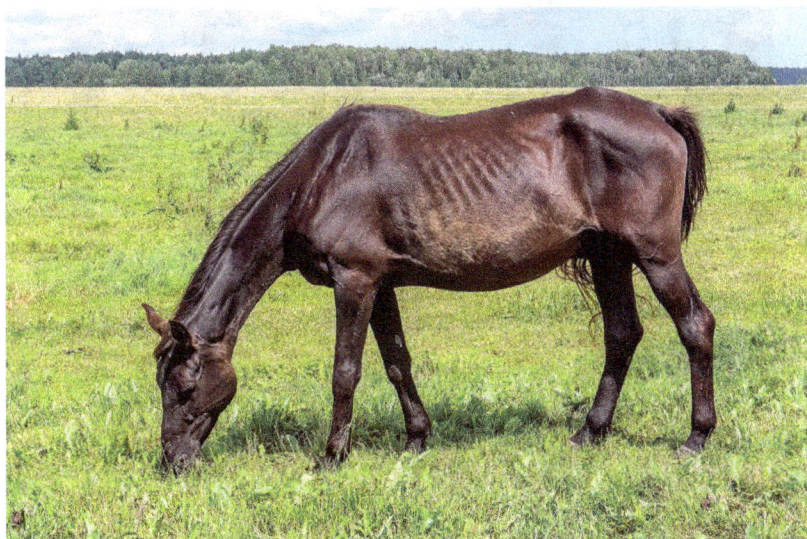

Figure 3.3 For good, healthy average condition, you should be able to feel your horse's ribs but not see them, unless he is turning away from you. This horse is obviously too thin, which could be due to several reasons, most commonly insufficient food for the horse's lifestyle and work, exposure to bad weather, digestive problems or parasite/worm infestation. Teeth in poor condition also prevent the horse processing his food adequately, whether grass, hay or other feeds.
Source: (Shutterstock ID: 1060669688)

do on a first aid basis for injuries or illnesses, it is obviously good sense to go along with your vet's advice. A short warning story:

Some years ago, as a freelance teacher, I had a new client to teach who was obviously taking all her advice from her fellow livery clients, the yard on which they kept their horses not having an experienced, knowledge-able equestrian manager but being simply a DIY yard renting out boxes. One day I arrived and she told me she had just found her horse lame in the field and brought him in. She could not have her lesson, clearly, and had rung the vet. The vet duly arrived and diagnosed a slight tendon sprain, the treatment comprising inflammatory medicine and several days' box rest.

Box rest, of course, means that a horse has to stay in the box for 24 hours of every day to rest the injury, but as soon as the vet had left the owner put a sheet on her horse and a headcollar, which I watched somewhat puzzled, and proceeded to bring him out of his box. I tactfully

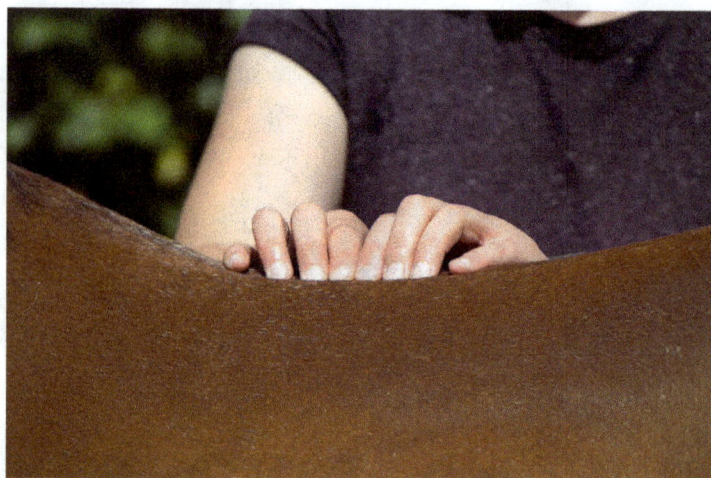

Figure 3.4 Acupressure is a therapy obviously related to acupuncture, and it is possible for owners to learn basic techniques from a practitioner willing to demonstrate. Formal courses are also available and can be found via the internet.
Source: (Shutterstock ID: 1447801103)

(I think!) asked her what she was doing and she looked at me as though I were stupid, answering 'Turning him out again, obviously.' I checked that she knew exactly what 'box rest' meant – in the box all the time. She had not understood that, but said 'Oh, I'm not doing that to him. He wants to be out.' I offered the advice that he needed to be in on a low-energy diet, plenty of hay, water and good bedding, and that if she turned him out he would be galloping around with his friends and making his lameness worse.

It was all to no avail. She turned him out and I heard from another client at that yard that he did, indeed, seriously lame himself to the point that he was, this time, standing on three legs. Apparently, the vet came on a continuing basis to treat the horse and he ended up spending several weeks on box rest rather than a few days, and suffered not only the boredom of being in all the time but also not a little pain in his leg as a consequence of his owner ignoring her vet's advice. The owner, of course, was saddled with expensive veterinary costs and was unable to ride her horse for several weeks because she ignored her vet's advice. In cases like that, permanent lameness can result and she was fortunate that that did not happen to her horse.

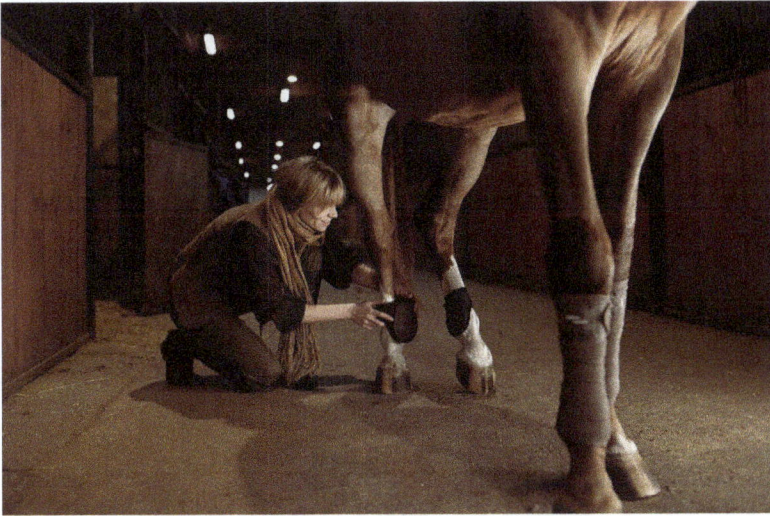

Figure 3.5 There are many forms of leg protection for horses, but wrongly chosen or applied, they can create injuries rather than protecting the legs. Commonly, boots and bandages are fitted too tightly, interfering with the function of the tendons and ligaments. Conversely, leg protection applied too loosely is not only useless but also dangerous if it shifts sufficiently to interfere with a horse's action. Tension and pressure can be difficult to gauge, but a lesson from a professional can be a great help.
Source: (Courtesy Alamy)

Euthanasia is an issue most of us don't like to think about, but it is something that can always face us, no matter how young or old our horse is. No vet would advise that a horse be put down if he or she did not seriously think it was necessary and the kindest thing to do in the circumstances. Those circumstances can vary from incurable, painful illness or injury through old age, loss of owner's income, an owner leaving the country or losing interest in horses and various other reasons.

The question to ask ourselves is: if the horse is *not* put down, what will happen to him? Considerations to think about are, can he expect a happy, future life in another home if he is sold as, say, a companion or for 'gentle hacking'? Could he find a home in a refuge such as an equestrian or general animal charity to live out his life there or, depending on the charity's policy, be rehomed while still belonging to the charity (and so having annual checks on his welfare)? There are many reasons for owner and horse having to part company, and most of us would want to find a

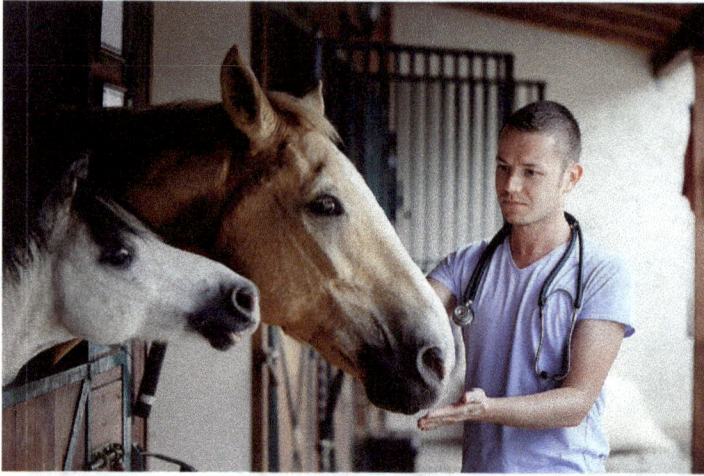

Figure 3.6 If you have a box or pen large enough (ideally twice the size of a normal box), two friends are often happier living together. Happiness is a great health boost for any species. With sensitive training and handling, living together does not automatically cause two equine friends to be almost impossible to separate.
Source: (Shutterstock ID: 1966382617)

good home for a horse we can no longer keep, whether by selling him or giving him away, in either case ideally to someone we know and trust to look after him properly. Equine and animal charities can play a large part in helping your horse, either by taking him in themselves or finding him another home.

If it comes to it and you cannot find a solution, I believe the horse's situation should be discussed in detail with the horse's vet. If it is determined that the only safe option for, say, an old, badly injured or permanently sick or lame horse is to euthanise him or her, what should we do? I firmly believe that it is an owner's duty, in such a case, not to allow the horse to be taken away while he or she is still alive but, upsetting though this is, to be with him throughout the procedure, carried out at home, and for the owner to gain the vet's assurance that the horse is, indeed, dead. Most commonly today euthanasia is carried out by means of the injection of a lethal drug rather than shooting. It is fine to leave then rather than see the horse's body winched into the wagon and removed.

If you cannot bear any of this, it is understandable but, for the horse's sake, ask a trusted friend the horse knows and likes to be with him

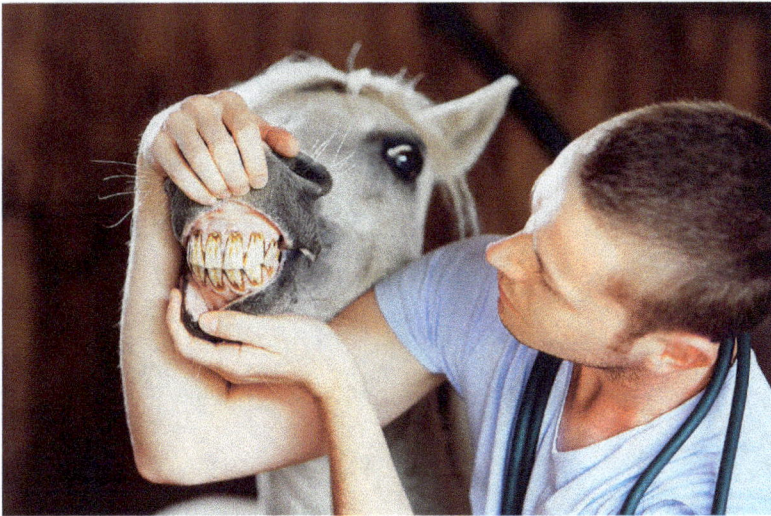

Figure 3.7 Horses' teeth should not be out of sight, out of mind. Healthy teeth, which 'fit' together in the right way and are regularly (every six months) inspected by an equine dentist or vet, make a massive difference to a horse's comfort, contentment and health. The back teeth (molars) in particular, because the upper jaw is a little wider than the lower one, wear to razor sharpness on the inner edges of the lower molars and the outer edges of the upper ones, making eating painful and wounding the cheeks and tongue. This unfortunate evolutionary feature is a frequent cause of death in feral horses, who ultimately starve, especially if they eventually reach the point where they cannot even close their mouths due to the overgrowth of enamel.
Source: (Shutterstock ID: 695133184)

if at all possible, and confirm with the vet that the horse is, indeed, dead and is not going to 'come round' before he is taken away. This may seem unnecessary but I have done it with my own horses and no vet has ever given the impression that he or she thought I was being over the top. It gives you complete peace of mind, knowing that your horse has been treated kindly and professionally, and is not going to be seen weeks later in an auction ring for sale. This seems to happen more times than you would believe. I confess to never having been to a slaughterhouse but have been told that the atmosphere of fear, the smell of blood, the strange people and unfamiliar surroundings greatly frighten the animals, of whatever species, and I would not want that for any animal of mine.

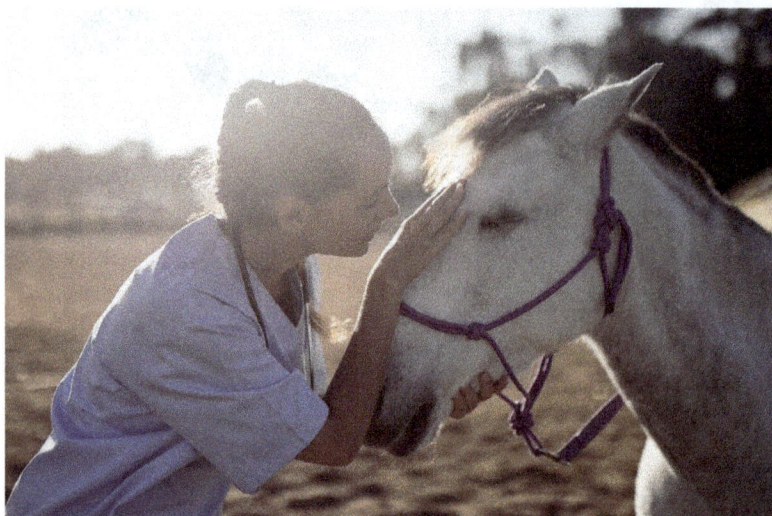

Figure 3.8 In these competitive days, it is extremely common for people to have horses only or mainly because they want to compete with them or follow a sport such as hunting. A horse is fortunate if his owner keeps him because they love the horse, not merely because of what the horse can do for them. I know that horses can tell the difference, too, between being loved and being used.

Source: (Shutterstock ID: 728128093)

3.6 GENERAL CONSIDERATIONS REGARDING HEALTH AND WELL-BEING

We have to accept that many people involved with horses regard them as commodities to be used. While many of us do not like this attitude, if the horse is well-treated he will, in practice, if owned and handled by experienced horse people with correct principles regarding animal welfare in general, be much better off than in the hands of someone who, through lack of training and experience in the right ways to manage horses, actually, often unknowingly but not always, treats him poorly. Loving a horse, as many of us do, is certainly not enough to maintain him in the manner to which he should be accustomed! Any horse will thrive and be much happier and, yes, healthier if his owner takes the trouble to find out how to properly look after horses and not leave every decision to, say, a livery yard owner who may or may not be an experienced horse person or hold the right values as to their care and entitlements.

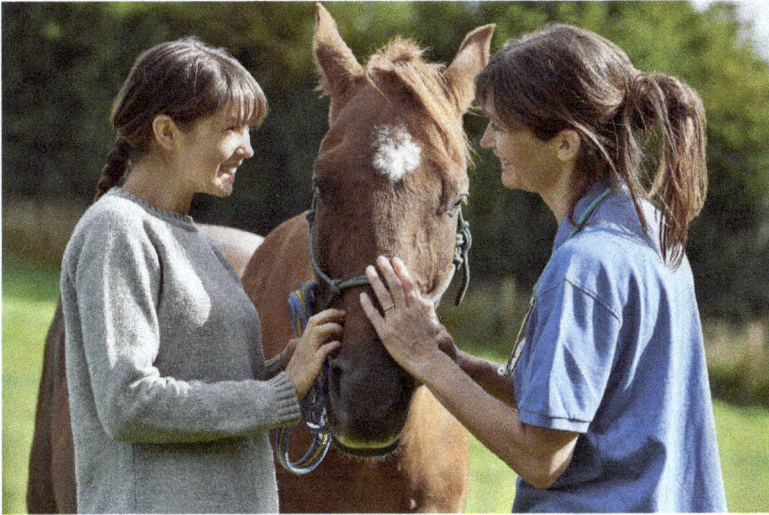

Figure 3.9 If at all possible, always be present yourself when your horse has to have any kind of treatment. If your relationship is good, your presence will reassure him and make the whole process potentially less stressful. Having said that, modern vets seem to me to be much more tuned in to horses' feelings than some were decades ago. Veterinary attention is expensive these days, but a vet who can instantly form good relations with their patients is worth his or her weight in gold – if not literally!

Source: (Courtesy Alamy)

These days, social media is often people's first port of call when information or advice is needed, yet social media must be the biggest source of mis-information ever invented judging by some of the posts one can read there. Just because someone owns a horse, it does not mean they know how to look after him properly. Buying a horse does not involve necessary training or an examination to qualify to take on the health and welfare of a sensitive, living creature (which applies to any living creature, of course).

Horses are sensitive animals, a point which can be belied by their size and strength, and, from a health point of view which is the subject of this part of the book, they do not thrive if not given conditions that make them content, confident, comfortable, happy and secure. It is not going too far to suggest that horses *expect* certain aspects of treatment, such as the provision of food, the presence of other horses and, I feel, decent

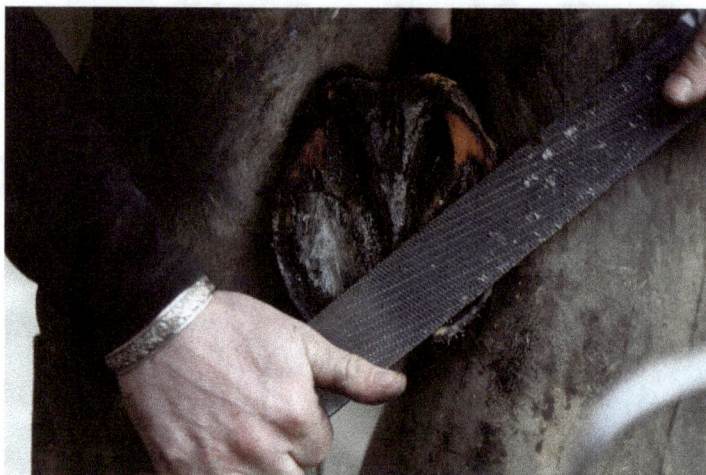

Figure 3.10 Whether your horse is shod or goes barefoot, the services of a good farrier are essential to his comfort and health. Shoeing a horse in front only, usually for economy, is a misguided practice because horses move by pushing themselves along with their hind legs (and feet) more than pulling forward with the forelegs, whose main job is weight-bearing. The hind feet therefore come in for more pressure and wear than is often realised. Uncomfortable, even painful, hind feet are a frequently unrecognised cause in such horses of reluctance to work and of apparent or actual lameness. If we school horses correctly, we try to strengthen them gradually to bring a little more weight on to the hindquarters, and the feet of course, so lightening the forehand. Therefore, it is clearly crucial that the hind feet are properly protected.

Source: (Shutterstock ID: 2149536685)

treatment from humans. Even if people use horses for their living or the bestowing of prestige, they still, I firmly believe, have a duty to look after them well and appropriately as fellow living beings.

The equestrian industry and world in general now has multiple sources of excellent, qualified, professional help and advice, some of which has to be paid for. There are professional organisations for just about every aspect of horse care and riding, and I have no hesitation in advising those with queries or concerns to contact them (some of which are given at the end of this book) in order to get trustworthy help and advice. Social media may first be used to get a variety of ideas and an overview of what others think about your problem or query, but reliable back-up is certainly needed in many cases by speaking to the people who really know.

On health issues, I would certainly recommend that you contact your veterinary practice before any other source. Surely we all owe this to our horses, who are, in effect, prisoners of the human race, who, when well-treated, seem all too willing to be with us, work for us and to show us affection in many cases where trust has been established.

Horses' health and well-being can easily be affected by many aspects of our use of their talents and their willingness, whether that be travelling, competing, training, working and playing, breeding, buying and selling. One thing is certain – an unhealthy horse is a liability to us and our bank balances. It could involve cruelty to deprive a horse of appropriate treatment even if those who have charge of him on a daily basis do not recognise that something is wrong and needs attention. The work we ask horses to do for us is athletic work demanding a reasonable level of fitness, and it is potentially dangerous if we are using public roads a good deal, jumping, galloping or asking any other athletic effort from them. It actually pays to learn as much as we can from correct, reliable sources and to ask for help from knowledgeable people. The rewards, in every way, are priceless.

Behavioural Interactions

Four

4.1 RESTRICTION, TWO SIDES OF THE COIN

We have mentioned earlier that horses are by nature creatures of wide, open spaces. We all know this, but we are so used to seeing them confined in stables and still, sometimes, tethered in stalls that we don't give this natural lifestyle priority in the way we think about our horses and ponies.

It is true that horses are also very adaptable, a quality that has enabled them to survive to the present day in large numbers, if mainly in domestic conditions. They adapt to being stabled 24/7 in certain circumstances such as illness or injury but also various conveniences for their human owners: I hope, though, that most people will admit that this is not the best way to keep healthy horses. Most owners try their best to give their horses at least a few hours a day having some time off from work and out of their stables. We are all used to seeing how horses perk up at the prospect of going out into 'the field', by far preferably with a friendly companion. We also can't miss their desire to come in during bad weather! This, though, can be modified if there is reasonable shelter in their field, either a shelter-shed ideally with a stock of hay or haylage in it so that they have the best of both worlds, or dense tree cover, or an overgrown hedge between them and the prevailing wind and rain. Much depends on their breed, and it is the 'finer' breeds such as, especially, Thoroughbreds and most Arabians that make the most use of available shelter. A comfortable, well-fitting rug can greatly help such horses to bear adverse weather conditions but is not a complete substitute for a sound, roomy, well-supplied shelter-shed or, of course, being brought in to an inviting stable with clean, cushioning bedding, food and water.

A friend and I used to keep our horses at a farm with a new, large livery yard diversification. The farm owners had their own half-dozen or so horses and ponies which were turned out separately from the liveries. The livery horses were turned out and brought in at different times during the day according to their owners' schedules, but the farm owners'

DOI: 10.1201/9781003396376-5

horses invented their own schedules depending almost entirely on the weather. The shelter facilities in the fields were poor to moderate, and the farm horses were out together in a 'gang' on a different part of the farm from the liveries. The reason was that the family did not want any possible safety problems arising from their livery clients if they and their horses interacted with the family's horses. Fair enough, we all thought. There was no favouritism as such but also a, to my mind, risky practice created by the farm horses themselves, all the horses being stabled in inter-connected, converted barns with good indoor loose boxes so there were at most times livery owners and sometimes their children on the yard and in the stables area.

If the weather, at any time of year, was bland enough for the farm horses to be happy to stay out they did so. If the weather, summer or winter, became very uncomfortable – such as too many insects or hot sun in summer or bitter cold, excessive rain or snow in winter – they all came cantering down to the field gate, whichever field they were in, looking expectantly towards the buildings for someone to let them through and into their comforting stables. I say let them through because that was all that happened: they were not haltered and led in but charged through the opened gate down the track to the stable yard at a going-on canter, skidding into the yard and each finding their way into their own stables.

Any owners who happened to be around in the yard or stable blocks at the time were notified when the farm horses arrived at their gate, so that liveries could be safely stabled if tied up in the gangways for grooming or whatever, and children moved to safety until all was settled. In would trot the farm horses, each making his or her way to the open door of their loose box, where there would be hay or haylage waiting, clean beds, checked water and so on. Each horse found its own stable, went in and immediately started eating whatever was on offer, unless they decided to have a good roll first. When their doors were safely bolted, the livery horses' and owners' routines recommenced.

Unfortunately, one day, the gate to the farm horses' field had 'come open' and the horses found their own way down the track to the stables. You might think that there would be mayhem as the horses entered the yard and stable barns but, amazingly, they stopped at the open main door to the barns and waited to be 'given permission' (it seemed) before entering and finding their boxes.

The reason we left that yard was because it became the habit for the farm family to leave the gate to their horses' field open and allow their horses to come and go whenever they wished. Naturally, we thought, sooner or later there was going to be an accident – and, to be sure, there was a minor accident which could have been a lot more serious. A new livery horse was tied up at the end of a gangway, his owner out of sight in the tack room. The farm horses came in and, despite walking calmly to their boxes, knocked against the new horse who became frightened and, being tied up, nearly fell, which would have resulted in him swinging by the head on his lead rope. Thankfully, this did not happen.

When my friend's and my horses were tied up in the gangways we never left them, but one day, my friend went to the tack room to fetch something she had forgotten. I happened to come out of my horse's box during the five minutes she was missing and, to my horror, found a toddler sitting on the ground immediately behind her horse's hind feet. The toddler was the child of a new owner who had just arrived on the yard and admitted that she knew little about horses apart from having ridden at a riding school. She had been warned not to let her child wander freely but took no notice as she 'wanted him to get used to horses'! I called to her to come and get her child NOW which, thankfully, she did, but this incident, plus because of the increasingly lax attitude of the farm family to the propensities of horses as opposed to cattle, and the different ways of managing and handling them, and their tendency to treat our horses like cows, we felt it safer to leave.

Horses are not stupid, of course, and they adapt remarkably well to the differing lifestyles and handling methods we equestrians believe to be best for us and them, but, like so many things in life, it is a case of 'everything in moderation' when caring for our horses. We need to be as adaptable towards them as we expect them to be towards us and, with their known physical and psychological qualities and needs, it seems to me that they are far more willing to adapt than we humans! Some horses can live out all the time depending on available facilities, but some can't. Horses, like humans, don't get on with all their kith and kin but have preferences as to which other horses they can and will get on with. Feeding, of course, is very individual and serious, even fatal, illnesses can arise from feeding which is faulty for a particular individual. We need to consider all possibilities when planning a care routine for our horses, or choosing a potential home for them, to establish as well as possible what will suit each individual. Thankfully, the basics are the same – all horses need appropriate food, water, shelter, freedom and exercise, and, with very rare exceptions, company.

Animals are as prone to stress disorders as are humans, but we probably have the advantage of knowing how to alleviate our stress, or at least understanding what is causing it whether we can improve our situation or not. Speaking generally, most horses adapt well to being stabled – a situation which is completely unnatural to their species: just because a foal may be born in a stable does not mean he or she will automatically adapt to a life without freedom. Even horses who, from birth, spend a good deal, or most, of their daily hours in a stable, relish freedom and close, tactile company. I feel it is gross bad management, cruel even, to prevent a horse exercising himself at will in a paddock or field and to deny him the company of his own kind – and this kind of management is rife today, passed off as being the safest way to keep, for instance, valuable horses in case of 'accidents'.

In my time as a professional equestrian writer, I have been commissioned by magazines to visit many different kinds of establishments, in the UK and Ireland, and have cared for several horses, my own and other people's, of different breeds and types, in widely differing circumstances, and am convinced, after decades of doing so, that we cannot ignore the basic 'equine spirit', for want of a better expression – the need for near-constant availability of food, growing or hand-delivered, the natural interaction in freedom with other equines and the confidence and reassurance of feeling safe.

This does not mean that I believe in turning out entire male horses willy-nilly with mares of all ages and sizes and letting them mate indiscriminately as they might in the wild. Of course not. But I do feel it is essential that the three main principles of equine well-being, welfare even, of Friends, Freedom and Foraging must be provided if we have any interest at all in the ethics of having, owning or 'using' horses. As the heading to this section of the book indicates, there are two sides to the coin – total freedom and total restriction. In domestic conditions, total freedom is not possible unless you are going to turn your horse on to the nearest moorland and leave him to fend for himself (as has happened in certain areas of the UK during the current, ongoing financial crisis). Total restriction happens far more than, I believe, it should or needs to in many different types of equestrian establishments.

Horses certainly appreciate being able to come in to comfortable accommodation with all their needs catered for. They also love being able to experience freedom, foraging for food and interacting with friends. Surely, it is our responsibility to provide them, in the massive majority of cases, with both.

4.2 EQUINE BEHAVIOURAL EXPRESSION

It always surprises me how many people think that horses do not have expressive faces. And how many misjudge a horse's real feelings which, of course, can be dangerous. Horses use their whole bodies to express their feelings from their muzzles to their tails, including their actions and general demeanour. Let's consider the most common, and important, gestures and postures of horses to get a better idea of what emotions a horse is trying to express.

Happiness and sadness. of the two, probably happiness is the easiest to 'read'. A happy horse is fairly calm but can be quite animated. He will have an enquiring look about his face, his eyes open and bright and his ears pointed towards anything interesting. His muzzle, comprising his nose, lips and chin area, is sensitive and expressive as it is used to smell, feel and taste food and other things which might be of interest. If the nostrils are partly closed rather than wide and 'flaring' (circular) but the horse is clearly paying attention to something, whether us, his feed, what's going on outside or in the distance, the nostrils will be mobile and he may snort as he both sends messages and draws in smells to give himself more information about his surroundings.

His body will be between relaxed and tense, depending on what is catching his attention, and his tail may be comfortably and loosely laid between his buttocks. He may whicker to us or another animal nearby, but basically, happiness, particularly when it is the horse's normal state of being (in which case congratulate yourself on providing circumstances that make him so), varies between alertness and calmness but indicates a normally healthy, content horse.

Sadness is as heartbreaking for a horse as it can be for us. Although horses and most other animals do not cry in the way we do, their facial expressions can show their emotional pain by being tense, their eyes may be sunken, the horse will have lower interest than usual in his surroundings and stand with his poll level with or lower than his withers, and have a dejected look about him. Sadness can certainly be felt by horses: it can be caused mainly by the absence, for a short or long time, of a close friend and, if longer term, can cause a horse to go off his feed. It is possible for a vet to give a horse a quick pick-me-up to help him overcome his sadness, but basically, if the cause of his sadness cannot be overcome, simply be with him as much as you can, treat him kindly and try to ensure another amiable companion for him.

Calmness and excitement. Calmness can be shown by simply a peaceful aura conveying a feeling of security and confidence. The horse will be interested in his environment, with ears pricking towards anything interesting, but generally he will be self-contained and have an air of confidence about him. Excitement also can exude confidence, but the horse will be animated, ears pricked, nostrils mobile and maybe he will be snorting. He may toss his head, paw the ground with his forefeet, have a raised tail and may even be whinnying at whatever he is excited about, provided he is not actually frightened (see later).

Sleepiness or alertness. Horses can doze heavily while standing up. Their poll will probably be lower than their withers, their eyes either closed or half so, maybe the bottom lip will droop and the horse will be resting a hind leg. He will change the leg occasionally. His tail will be loose and hanging still. Alertness, on the other hand, means he is more than just awake, but is taking particular notice of some sight, sound or smell nearby or not too far away. His ears, the eternal messengers, will be pricked towards whatever is interesting him. It is possible for one ear to be forward while the other is back, as he scans all around him.

Fear versus confidence and security. Fear is a dangerous emotion in horses for humans, and for the horse himself. Horses often act without thinking when frightened, more so than humans do. The eyes will be wide open, maybe showing their whites, the whole face will be tense, the nostrils rounded to take in information via smell, the ears directed, forward or back, towards whatever is frightening the horse, and the tail will be raised with a stiff dock. If the object of fear is behind the horse, his tail may instead be clamped between his buttocks in a protective way and his ears will be pointed backwards, as well. Conversely, confidence and security are shown by a steady appearance, interest in what is ahead, whether it is an obstacle, a familiar route or the gate to Home! He will move confidently and straight towards the object of his interest.

Jealousy is an emotion we do not normally think much about in connection with horses. I once kept a horse at a yard where a friend also kept his horse, at the other end of the row of boxes. I would exercise his horse as well as mine some days depending on his working hours. It was a good livery yard and I was fortunate that the owner would help me out and go into my horse's box, pretending to be needing to do something with him, while I got out of the yard on my friend's horse, which stopped mine kicking the living daylights out of his stable door because I was riding another horse! Once home again, I dismounted before entering the yard and sneaked my friend's horse back into his box before mine could see us – but he could smell him on my clothes and was not too happy!

So far as jealousy between horses is concerned, this can, indeed, cause injuries if fights occur between horses because one of them does not want other horses near his friend, for example. For this reason, relationships between horses must be closely watched regularly to ensure that all horses who have free access to each other, such as when they are turned out together, agree and do not have arguments which could result in injury. (Here I would stress that there is little danger of friendly horses injuring each other. Injuries in such a case are a very poor excuse for owners not allowing horses to enjoy close, tactile contact with their friends. What about the mental harm of horses not being allowed friendships? That is just as important.)

Anger. There are few more emotions as frightening as seeing an angry horse, except perhaps one that is frightened out of its wits with fear and is not thinking straight. When a horse is angry, his attention is focussed entirely on whatever it is that he is angry about and a horse, believe it, can very easily kill a human within reach. What sort of thing makes a horse angry? It may be something as simple as another horse he really dislikes, or, of course, a human who perhaps smells of such a horse, or simply with an aroma the horse really dislikes. It may be that someone is doing something to the horse that he hates, such as rough grooming, dousing him with cold water or teasing him with his feed, none of which a true horseman or horsewoman would dream of doing to a horse.

(Back in the 1980s, I visited a military yard to write an article about their horses, and was horrified to see the soldiers tie up their horses in the yard, once home, and turn the fire hoses on them to clean them up, as they were very muddy after work. The horses clearly did not like this one bit, as you would expect, but the soldiers thought it was funny. I couldn't believe my eyes. I asked a nearby officer if that was normal procedure and, with a smug smile on his face, he said it was. It was an excellent way of cooling down hot horses, he said, and of getting rid of mud. The soldiers had enough to do already without using more conventional methods of getting their horses clean again, he said. I put this in my article, along with my 'anti' comments. The editor printed the facts, but,

I suppose understandably, deleted my criticisms. Actually, this is appalling horse management and, in my view, amounts to cruelty. I hope their practices have improved now.)

Pain. Horses show pain very clearly, but some people confuse it with anger (part of which can be involved). A horse in pain with colic, say, will be restless, pacing his box, usually snatching at his sides, getting up and down and rolling frequently. Other internal pain may be shown by the horse standing tensely, perhaps with a raised spine and an anxious look on his face, nostrils drawn up and back, ears directed back towards the pain and his eyelids in a triangular shape which indicates anxiety. Sometimes a horse in pain will thrash his tail as well. Lameness, obviously, is clear in a horse's uneven action: his head will drop on the sound leg to take the weight off the painful one. It should be remembered that horses' feet can cause them pain: this can be due to, say, a stone being caught between the frog and the sole, a horse with flat feet working on rough going, or shoes being left on too long which interfere with the foot's normal functioning and unbalancing the normal stride.

People often do not recognise pain in a ridden horse when it is caused by bad riding (even in some purportedly expert riders using horse-unfriendly methods), and the cause can be badly fitting tack, badly adjusted tack, harsh whipping (which should never be carried out, the whip being used for tapping messages to a horse, never punishment), harsh use of reins and, therefore, bit, tack which is uncomfortable such as insufficient room around the base of a horse's ears, tight throatlatches and, very common today, nosebands so tight that the horse cannot even partially open his mouth to adjust the position of the bit, use it to send messages up the reins to his rider or use his tongue as part of the jaw action needed to swallow his saliva. This is given away by the presence of froth from the mouth. (A horse's mouth should never froth as such, but simply be comfortably moist to enhance a fair, gentle bit contact.) Tight nosebands can also cause the horse's cheeks to be cut on the edges of his teeth, and cause tongue injuries.

Even well-fitted saddles can cause problems if we put them on too far forward, as is common, so that the front of the saddle presses on and interferes with shoulder movement. It is quite possible for it to actually bruise the tops of the horse's shoulders when they move back and forth during foreleg action. Also, a saddle too far forward will naturally cause the girth to be too far forward as well, pressing into and bruising the space behind the horse's elbow. If the saddle is too far back, of course, it can bruise the loins. (Badly fitting rugs, too, can cause sustained soreness, pain and discomfort, worn as they are for several hours at a time.) A saddle pad is not the answer to a badly fitting or placed saddle as it will probably unbalance the saddle and cause problems generally.

Checking the fit of tack is not difficult. We should be able to *easily* pass a finger under all parts of a bridle including nosebands, and make sure the bottoms of the ears have plenty of clearance. The throatlatch should allow a sideways-on hand to be fitted between it and the horse's round jawbone and the noseband, like the rest of the bridle, should allow *at least* one finger, and preferably two or even three fingers, to be fitted between it and the horse's nasal bone down the front of his face. A finger should be able to be slid between any strap dropped into the curb/chin groove, and curb chains must be loose enough to lie in the groove, not above it.

4.3 IS IT OUR FAULT AND CAN WE HELP?

The fitting of tack and clothing is obviously an area in which we have full responsibility. We can help by fitting everything correctly and seeing that the horse is comfortable. Pain for other reasons may well need expert help in finding out exactly where and why a horse is showing signs of being in pain or, at least, not feeling very well. A very experienced horse person could well help, but I suggest we don't delay in calling out a veterinary surgeon to diagnose what is causing the condition if we really cannot deal with it ourselves, and what can be done about it. This is one of the unavoidable expenses involved in correct, humane horse care. Veterinary costs have sky-rocketed in recent years, not least because of the sheer expense of running a modern practice, wages, equipment costs that cannot be passed on to clients via bills, drugs the cost of which can, running vehicles and all the myriad expenses involved in a professional practice.

Insurance costs are also sky-high and many people simply cannot afford adequate insurance for their horses. A common plan is to get quotes from several companies, calculate an average and save that amount every month into a savings account especially for veterinary and other health expenses. This seems to work well for many people unless a really expensive, serious condition arises, in which case a horse will need simply to be put down. Thankfully, this is a rare event, except for those owners who regard their horses as long-term, family members and know they are going to have to face it one day anyway.

It might sound like a callous thing to say, but, within reason, if we cannot afford to keep a horse well and healthy, whether or not he or she is working, perhaps we should be thinking of somehow rehoming him, perhaps with a friend, maybe on a share basis with a trusted horse-lover or, if the horse is elderly or cannot work, seeing if an equine charity could adopt him. Horses are helpless when it comes to situations like this and we really do have a responsibility to ensure their health and happiness. Not only is it good for the horse but also it makes us feel better, having done the right thing by our horse.

4.4 INTERACTIONS WITH HUMANS, HORSES AND OTHER SPECIES

Horses are, of course, very social animals and interact freely, when allowed and given the opportunity, with animals of other species, also making animal friends, just as we do. It would be wonderful to really know how they think of us! If they think of us as simply another kind of animal, I wonder what they make of our treatment and training of them. Do they understand that we think we are their bosses, or at least friends or do they think of us as other animals who do things with them, provide food and control their lives? Sadly, we can't speak Horse to the extent to which we could ask them.

We discussed earlier how horses express their feelings and they use this very same system to communicate with us as well as with other horses and animal species. So, we do have to familiarise ourselves with horses' language to understand how they are feeling and maybe what they are planning to do.

I was once in the stable with a horse I had recently bought and who had a reputation for being 'difficult', a description which turned out to mean actually 'dangerous'! A few years earlier, I had had a great deal of success with a mare who bit everyone freely if she didn't like them, and transformed her simply with fair but firm treatment and sensible behaviour when I was with her. I took no chances: she was well known for biting people, her go-to form of expression for anyone new or suspect, so I thought I was going to have the same success with my new, dangerous horse. Foolish woman! To cut a long story short, he was a one-person horse. When I was the only person dealing with him (he was at a do-it-yourself livery) he appeared to be a transformed character, but when more than one person was involved with him, he tried to savage all except the one who had most to do with him.

After a couple of months, I was ill and could not go to care for him, so the yard owner bravely took him over. He was a saint with her because no one else dared to do him, so when I returned to duty I found that he

Behavioural Interactions

had transferred his affections to the yard owner and jilted me. For some reason, he did not transfer his trust back to me. One day, he cornered me in his box by backing into a corner when I was skipping out and threatening me with his hind feet whenever I moved. I had a paper bag in my pocket with Mint Imperials in it, thank heaven, so I slowly downed tools, rustled the bag in my pocket, got it out and started noisily chomping a mint. He could not resist turning to see what was going on: as he turned his head round to the right I nipped up his left side and out of his door. By the time he had turned back with an amazed look on his face, I was outside with the door safely bolted. I then went to find the yard owner, describing what had happened and asking her to take him over again.

Not long after that, I gave up as he clearly no longer wanted me, and I gave him to a friend who got on with him like a house on fire. She left her coat hanging outside his box one night and the next morning found that he had brought it into his box and slept on it. Every night after that, she left her coat there and he brought it in, presumably because it smelled of her and he felt close to her. Horses!

So – our interactions with our horses involve our learning and understanding their messages, expressions and actions. But they use exactly the same language to us as to horses and other animals. I have always found that horses are quite happy in the company of other species of animal, whether in the field, out hacking or in their stable. Cats, in particular, seem to like resting on the backs of stabled horses and I used to know one horse who would wander about the yard and field with the stable cat on his back, both of them quite happy to be together.

The first time I managed to hack out my first horse with my dogs – a fond dream I had had for years – I found he disliked the dogs and they never stopped barking at him and jumping up at my legs, really annoying him, so I had to cut short the ride and give up on that dream. However, when he was turned out the dogs and he would loaf about in the field quite unconcerned at each others' presence, although not exactly friendly.

Horses readily make friends with people, other horses and other animals, including birds. Interestingly, they do use exactly the same physical signals described earlier to all of them and seem to be able to learn the other species' languages, too, which I think is remarkable. Where does that leave us? We know they learn our vocal languages and body language, for example. When lungeing horses or working them loose, they quickly learn our physical signs such as a raised hand or arm, our bending down to slow them, stand level with their hip to speed them up, and so on. If we are consistent, a most important quality to horses, they soon learn our way of communicating with them and, in a working situation such as working loose, they watch us all the time and very quickly indeed learn our body language, seeming, in my experience, to enjoy working with us in this way.

I do feel that we under-estimate horses' abilities to communicate with us, their desires readily to have a 'conversation' with us and, who knows, to me they seem to actually *expect* us to communicate with them. They all like working loose with us, I find, except one mare I had who felt, by all her body language and attitude, that it was of no interest and maybe even below her to play humans' games like that! Mares, like cats versus dogs, feel, I am sure, more superior than male horses whether stallions or geldings. In the wild or rather, today, feral environments, a stallion is only a lodger and is dismissed from the family herd as they wish by the mares.

My old Thoroughbred mare mentioned earlier was a former racehorse and the head lad at her livery yard when she came to me was a former head lad on racing yards – they got on like cream on peaches! When I could not get to the yard to take her out or do her, he would long-rein her around the village, but, eventually, she decided the route, noted all the shops where she got tit-bits and told him which way they were going, deciding when she wanted to go home. If it was raining she would not leave her box.

In that same village, decades earlier when life was slower and less hampered round and about by all sorts of rules and regulations, there was an elderly gelding whose name I forget, who made many human and canine friends. His (male) 'owner' used to walk him *loose* around the village and he just toddled along following him, but stopping at every shop or house where he knew he would get a treat or even just a fuss. He would actually go into the shops, talk in his way to the shop owners who fed him mints and other sweeties, then 'rein back' out and down the steps as there was never room for him to turn round, and off he would go to the next shop. At houses, he would stand outside and look hopefully through the window for a minute or two, waiting for someone to come out and give him a tit-bit. If it didn't materialise he would just go along to the next stopping point. When he wanted to go home again, he 'told' his owner who had to go along with what the horse wanted. Imagine that happening today!

Horses are far more intelligent than we imagine, I do know that. They are very willing to be friends, to interact with us on an equal inter-species basis and expect us to understand them. It really isn't difficult if we try. I find it so upsetting to see how harshly horses are used by many people today. They are bossed about as though they are underlings just there to do as they are told, when their humans could have so much better a relationship with them if they treated them more kindly and equally, but maybe the humans do not want that. Horses' strength, speed and jumping ability act as a real power-kick for many people, especially those who are competitive, it seems, but even so, it is not necessary to browbeat them, subjugate them and treat them as tools for glory and prestige.

Thousands of horses every year, just in the UK, are put down just because they can no longer work, some of them quite young, but there are not, it appears, enough homes to give a secure and loving future to all horses who are unwanted simply because they could not run fast enough, jump high enough or were not strong or agile enough for whatever task their human had planned for them. It is true that euthanasia must be better than a future life being passed from pillar to post, hand to hand, and quite possibly experiencing inadequate care, because they were part of the surplus thousands of youngsters bred every year to make money but were unable to come up to some human's requirements for them. Here in the UK, we do not knowingly eat horse flesh, so we do have a problem with excess numbers of unwanted horses, and at the time of writing we might still send them abroad for the continental meat market although this should change in the very near future.

4.5 GIVING HORSES CHOICES IN THEIR LIFESTYLE

When we look at the lifestyle of truly feral horses we can see that they do not have great variety – they eat for very roughly 14 hours a day depending on the quality of their food, they sleep for a few hours, roughly six hours, they spend the rest of their time interacting with their herd mates, dozing or napping and the least time galloping away from any predators or dealing with other 'nuisance' animals, including humans.

Compare, or rather contrast, this with the lifestyle of a domesticated, working horse. For most of his time he will be stabled, probably for at least the length of time he would spend grazing and foraging in a feral lifestyle. He will, hopefully, have food, probably hay, with him in his box for much of that time (if he hasn't his digestive health and mental well-being are at risk), for, say, up to two hours most days he will be working or exercising and, again hopefully, for the remaining few hours he will be free with other horses. What a difference from the life he evolved to live!

It is true that feral horses do not live so long as domestic ones (bearing in mind that many of the latter are euthanised early in life) and their lives are stressful, especially in regions where they are susceptible to predation from carnivores. Feral horses also live a truly wild life in that they are at the full mercy of the natural phenomena of the weather and climate. This involves not only tolerating the effects of the weather on their bodies which is tough enough, but also their very food supplies are dependent on the weather as well, as to how well the grass and other vegetation grows, or doesn't.

Feral horses live in very varied areas of the world, from near-arctic conditions in Russia to the baking hot Namib Desert in Africa and all climates in between. It is also noticeable that in most natural areas where feral horses exist shelter from the rigours of the local climate seems to be very sparse. Horses and what we call ponies are very adaptable, but even they cannot overcome their natural physiology so far as climate resistance is concerned. Those whose ancestors evolved in cold areas have thicker skins and coats, plus resistance to cold while those originating in hot areas such as Arabia (although I understand that Arabia's climate can be quite variable) are geared to hotter environments, with thinner skins and coats.

Domestic horses and ponies may not have the freedom of choice of feral ones, but they are better protected from the weather, generally speaking. Unfortunately, this protection usually consists of confinement to a stable or other human construct. The luckiest domestic horses have accommodation offering both an open shelter and space to move about with others at faster gaits, which equines enjoy. The final finishing touch so far as accommodation is concerned is grass growing on the ground.

In the latter case, the horses have a good choice of where to be and whether or not they can spend much of their time, as they would in Nature, eating – either growing food or that provided by their carers.

How can we give them more lifestyle choices? As beings who have a good deal of choice over their lives, we must find it hard to imagine what it is like to be controlled, from 'being in prison' at one extreme to 'living a life of exposure to the elements' at the other. The ideal, I am sure the horses would confirm, is a half-way house solution – freedom and company with available shelter when needed, constituting better accommodation than most stabled and feral horses. And, really, it should not be that difficult to achieve. It is very difficult, when keeping horses at livery, to find truly horse-friendly accommodation for our equine loved ones, in my many years of livery experience, mainly because the livery yard owners are not willing to provide it even when they easily could. Horses are kept liberally all over our country, but it seems that genuinely horse-friendly yards are certainly in the minority.

What do I mean by a horse-friendly yard? Well, one that is designed and constructed, or adapted, to provide the facilities that horses really need in order to live the nearest possible domestic version, in most cases, to the life they evolved to live – the now-famous phrase Friends, Freedom and Foraging plus the advantages of shelter. Domestic horses of necessity have to be constrained within fenced areas, with the exception of some locations like the New Forest or moorland areas, but (almost) any turnout is better than none. A scientific survey a few years ago showed that horses' Number One priority was not lots of space to run around in but the presence of company. Apparently, the horses placed this requirement above that of the provision of food! How the research team determined this parameter I don't know, but it is not really surprising.

In domestic conditions, the most horse-friendly design or provision of accommodation for horses is a large shelter shed opening on to a surfaced area which will not become fetlock deep in mud in wet weather, opening again on to pasture with, ideally, plenty of natural shelter available as well. Company goes without saying as do the more or less constant provision of food (hay or haylage mostly) and a permanent, clean water supply, artificial or natural. (Many so-called natural supplies' of water in a survey some years ago were found to look crystal clear but were, in fact, contaminated by various pollutants, some of which could be very harmful.)

In conditions like those described, horses can be extremely happy as they have everything they could want. We see also the development, gradually, of more 'Paddock Paradises' for horses, where they have access to tracks to get them from paddock to paddock (opened and closed in turn as their grass is grazed down) with water sources in various places and gates opened or closed to allow access to various paddocks in use and to rest others. I have never been lucky enough to be able to use one of these, but one owner of such a facility rang me regarding a book and, as you do, we got talking and she told me all about her management. She was particularly impressed by the instant taking-on-board by the horses and ponies of which paddocks (gates) were open and which were not. When the time came to rest and treat particular paddocks, so closing them off and opening up rested ones for re-use, they were shown which gates were closed or open and remembered instantly where they could go and where they couldn't.

If you cannot come fairly close to something approaching large areas offering full and fairly natural facilities, or to a Paddock Paradise, how can you make your horse's life more what you would wish, more varied and horse-friendly? I know only too well how difficult really good livery is to find, livery that puts the horses first, that meets most of the horses' requirements, even all of them, and with a listening ear from the yard owner as to how things could be made even better if at all possible. It is also common to find livery yards owned by people who are willing to try to accommodate horses as they should live but have a modest knowledge, if any, of horses themselves. One such place I visited to teach had been a farm, purchased by a retired couple as an equestrian business to boost their lives and income in retirement, but with admittedly insufficient knowledge to effectively manage the place. Their solution was to offer free stabling, feed and everything else to a woman with two horses who really knew what was what where horses were concerned, to manage the horses' and their owners' requirements, which included coming down hard on those whose horse management left something to be desired. Another was a farmer who maintained a small herd of cattle for his interest but converted his buildings into loose boxes and a large indoor school. His land he turned over to growing hay for the horses – and turnips which they loved – selling the surplus. His two adult sons knew little about horses but were keen to learn the differences between equine and bovine requirements and, importantly, behaviour. I was impressed by their keenness and their willingness to provide what the owners wanted, and promptly, such as bringing round some more hay, mending a waterer that had gone on strike, operating a proper grazing rotation, buying a horse walker and so on. Unfortunately, places like those two are rare, in my experience.

The worst yards to be on are those with owners who are simply rent collectors, little or no horse knowledge and where there is not even a competent manager or 'in charge' horse owner. Welfare can be a major problem on yards like that, with no one able or willing to put things right. Sadly, there is still no legislation, so far as I can discover, to regulate livery yards even though there have been attempts to do so by concerned horse people over the years. The best that can be done is to contact an appropriate department (concerned with animal welfare) at your local council, or to report the yard to a charity, which may or may not be willing or able to help.

So, if you find yourselves on a yard leaving something to be desired, obviously start looking around for others, ask other owners, Google livery yards, in the UK ask the British Horse Society and the Association of British Riding Schools about their registers of livery facilities at riding schools or dedicated stables and generally keep your ears and eyes open. Some yards can be impossibly restrictive as to what you may and may not do, others are so free and easy as to be dangerous. You might be able to keep your horse with a friend or acquaintance who has their own facilities (although I would not be happy keeping a horse at a place with no living accommodation, that is, no one living there all the time and especially at night).

If you are on a yard that is mediocre but you would rather stay, you can always discuss with the owner what other facilities and/or services they could supply and whether or not they are willing and able to improve things. Consider changing your own routine, if possible, to enable you to lead your horse out to graze, for instance, or arrange with another competent owner to have your horse exercised free of charge if you help them with their stable work and you are able to do so. Ask around for additional grazing to rent, consider all your skills and see if you can use them to 'pay' for extra services and/or facilities for your horse. It is surprising how you can improve matters, with a little imagination and goodwill.

4.6 LEARNED HELPLESSNESS

This term means that a horse has learned that whatever he does he is helpless to improve his lifestyle. His normal equine reactions, such as the familiar flight-or-fight response, to escape stressful situations do not work as they are thwarted by his circumstances, including humans' actions, being tied up or fairly constantly stabled, often without sufficient occupation such as eating (one of the reasons we need to provide a fairly constant supply of appropriate hay) and without the amenable company or nearby presence of another horse.

Horses suffering from the depressed state of learned helplessness are usually inactive and dull as though they were ill, which in effect they are but mentally so. They have little interest in what is going on; some become sour in nature; others become prone to stereotypical behaviour (formerly called 'stable vices') such as crib-biting, wind-sucking, wood chewing or box walking; and others become vicious and dangerous. Sadly and shockingly, some trainers deliberately initiate this state to make horses obedient, calm and manageable. Many, perhaps more novice, people do not recognise the state and simply believe that the horse appears very well trained and behaved.

Learned helplessness can be very difficult to overcome. Badly affected horses do not improve much even when turned out with a friend because of the severe psychological effects on their brains, just as severe depression in humans rarely improves without professional treatment. However, it is not impossible to improve the condition and this can gradually be done by means of correct, sympathetic and accurately timed training methods and kind treatment, plus paying attention to the horse's needs as a horse – liberty, favoured company, ample and appropriate food, water and shelter. It is important to realise that the horse is not being disobedient or stubborn but that he is damaged and needs care and correct treatment. A conversation with your veterinary surgeon could be very enlightening to see whether medical intervention, as with human depressives, could help the horse.

Generally speaking, the practical ways to improve such a horse's condition are via training, riding and handling methods he understands and, here, the study of the elementary principles of Equitation Science will be invaluable. In conventional riding and training, we do not pay sufficient attention to the timing of our aids: in fact, instruction often asks us to 'keep doing something at every stride to keep your horse on the ball' whereas, in modern ES riding we stress that as soon as a horse has obeyed an aid we stop giving it so that the horse can connect his action with the reward of the aid stopping. This creates a light, interested, co-operative and confident horse. I have covered this topic very comprehensively in my book *Fine Riding* (CRC Press/Taylor & Francis). Other ways of helping such a horse include avoiding over-correction for 'mistakes' or misunderstandings and harsh treatment of any kind under any circumstances, incorporating variety in schooling sessions, hacking routes and so on, so that interest rather than boredom is created.

Of course, regular, preferably daily, turnout and social interaction with other horses, even only one friendly one, is the go-to cure for so many conditions. If turnout is not always possible, take the trouble to lead your horse around the place or off the yard if safe to do so, ideally with a well-behaved, friendly companion horse and his owner, to graze in hand. Most horses really enjoy this, and it also improves our own relationship with a horse. Horses do regard humans as company of a sort and soon work out who they like and who they don't, but another equine friend's company means a lot to any horse, particularly one with 'issues'.

4.7 LIMITATIONS ON BEHAVIOURAL EXPRESSION

This topic is very closely related to learned helplessness. It is crucial that we never approach the matter of training or controlling a horse to the point where he is browbeaten, except in rare situations of accident or illness when control for veterinary reasons is essential. Even here, older methods of control which could hurt or frighten horses are no longer approved of, and most veterinary surgeons, faced with applying uncomfortable or painful treatment to a horse, will readily give him a sedative, anaesthetic or whatever is necessary to calm a horse and avoid pain. Dealing with a horse involved in an accident is a skilled subject of its own and such a situation is best left to the professionals, although the presence of a self-controlled, sensible and preferably knowledgeable horseperson, ideally one the horse knows, can be a great comfort to him and a help to those trying to assist him.

For general purposes, it is perfectly possible, using the modern, scientifically proved techniques of Equitation Science, to train a horse humanely and extremely effectively, and I strongly recommend my readers to explore the websites of Equitation Science International (www.esi-education.com) and the International Society for Equitation Science (www.equitationscience.com). As mentioned earlier, my first book for CRC Press/Taylor & Francis, *Fine Riding*, gives a good deal of how-to information about Equitation Science (ES).

The massive majority of people prefer a horse's own personality to shine through but in a safe way. Horses who habitually bite, kick, rear, buck, run away and display similar dangerous behaviours have usually been badly treated and/or trained in the past. This does not necessarily mean that they have been whipped, spurred hard, had their mouths abused, been forced to work in painful tack or with sore feet and so on, although any of these can arise due to harsh or incomprehensible treatment. They can arise simply due to inexpert training/schooling involving insufficient *correctly-applied* training/control measures which have allowed or caused the horse to 'get away' with doing whatever he likes, or thinks best under his circumstances. Horses become frightened and defensive when they are confused, and this can certainly arise due to incomprehensible training methods, inconsistently applied aids, badly timed application and release of aids and, of course, being harshly treated in any way – a situation that can arise when an unknowledgeable 'trainer' is running out of ideas to 'get the horse to do it' (whatever it is) and resorts to 'a good hiding' or jabbing him in the mouth with the reins, and similar desperate measures which, I guarantee, will not improve the situation.

I am certain that most horses are of a co-operative nature and want to work, play and live with us in harmony. It is when things go wrong, nearly always due to horse-unfriendly training, handling and management methods, that they resort to self-defence if they possibly can. Unfortunately, some humans then sometimes get rough and tough with the horse which angers and/or frightens him or her. We apply restrictive gear to him, we start using the same aids that confused him in the first place but apply them with more pressure to 'keep him under control' (restrict his behavioural expression), so confusing and frightening or angering him even more, and the matter quickly escalates from bad to worse, becoming dangerous and upsetting for both parties. The horse's trust is damaged and horses have very long memories. Horses who are browbeaten and kept down are a sorry sight indeed. Some people confuse this state for good, calm behaviour.

Decades ago, there was a large troupe of Western cow ponies touring Britain, which attracted a good deal of attention wherever they appeared. Their human riders and handlers were all very open when asked questions, clearly proud of their horses and their accomplishments and seemed to be enjoying their visit to England. We British horse owners, all Riding Club members and well used to conventional, modern riding, watched their display of Western riding with some awe – the intricate and athletic movements of the horses in curb bits only and largely on a loose rein, the apparently huge saddles and the riders' seats and security – and were allowed to visit them in their temporary stables after their display. We noticed how quiet and detached the horses appeared in their stables. There was hay available but they were not eating it, people were everywhere but they largely ignored them, rather they were standing mostly at the backs of their boxes apparently in a world of their own. They did not look drugged, actually, but were, to us, unnaturally quiet. We had noticed during the display that each one or each small group came out and gave a very active display under their riders, then, when returned to the sidelines, just stood 'obediently' as though they knew every step of the display and were simply expecting their next task as part of a routine.

When we were looking around the stables, I commented to my friend that the horses were strangely quiet and looked as though they were bored with their job. In later years, with much greater knowledge of horse psychology, training and so on, I realised that every one of them was in learned helplessness (see earlier). Their display was perfect but, recalling their demeanour from all those years ago, it dawned on me that that was, indeed, the case. Just about every aspect of their behaviour was controlled, their personalities flattened, their spirits broken.

Today, when the horse world is so concerned about maintaining its Social Licence to Operate (SLO), I wonder how many horses, in reality, are suffering from learned helplessness and from having their behavioural expression squashed. Many horses working on the flat seem to me to be coerced into being ridden in a particular way that is, at present, regarded as how they should go, their riders appearing proud of this style and, worst of all, judges putting up competition horses presented in this way of going.

And what way of going is that? It is certainly, to me, an artificial way of going, with shortened necks, their heads held by their riders on the vertical but many also being presented behind the vertical and clearly uncomfortable. They show an exaggerated action, often have a defeated look in their eyes and froth excessively at the mouth – which indicates a cramped throat preventing them from swallowing their saliva, so it exits via the mouth as froth. And we still hear the old and erroneous view from Name riders that the more froth there is, the better. Absolutely not. It is extremely difficult to correct such situations when judges repeatedly put up and award championships to, I believe, unhappy horses ridden in such a restrictive way and unnatural posture or outline.

Jumping horses are allowed to go with much more freedom, even if their discipline has a dressage phase, but even here a close eye has to be kept on the jumping and galloping phases of the competition to ensure that the rider is not pushing his or her horse to the point of distress for the sake of winning. I do appreciate that it may be the rider's living that is at stake, but I have every hope that, in future, social pressure will bring about change for the better in athletic equestrian competition, and also in those disciplines that involve only flatwork, including endurance riding.

Horse racing of all types also has its critics and there is no doubt that horses can be pressured hard to win. Steps have been taken in recent years to protect the horses against, perhaps, some over-zealous riders, and the jumps the horses may have to negotiate have been modified.

With the rather slow but now relentless progress towards more humane methods of training, riding and presenting competition animals, and using horses and ponies for non-competitive riding activities such as hunting or even private hacking, equestrian sport is gradually learning that it is not immune from public criticism and it only takes one or two offenders who use their horses with insufficient care for their well-being and actual welfare to blacken the reputations of everyone else.

Most training of horses involves some element of limiting the horses' behavioural expressions, of course, but, training and riding with consideration and using methods understandable to the horse who, let's face it, cannot read his trainer's mind as to exactly what is expected of him, we should be able to be confident that equestrianism will continue in an improved format well into the future.

4.8 IDEAS FOR IMPROVING POOR LIVING CONDITIONS

It is easy for us to feel helpless as regards our horses' lives if we have to keep them in conditions we feel are not what we would like. In my long experience, good livery yards that have the horses' interests at heart are few and far between. They are mostly run as businesses, of course, and it is understandable that people fortunate enough to own land and associated buildings that permit them to operate a commercial livery yard, whether or not as part of a riding school, want and need to make a profit from the horses and their owners. This topic has been broached earlier, but next I give some ideas on what constitutes a good environment for horses, whether on a livery yard to perhaps give some encouragement to their owners, or on your own premises as your budget permits.

How big should a loose box be for, say, a 16hh/1.61m horse? The size of 12 feet square or 3.65 metre square has been quoted as being adequate, but I think this is minimal. As for height, the roof or ceiling should be high enough to not bang the horse on the head if he rears in his box. Perhaps the simplest way to work this out is to measure your horse from muzzle to dock and check that the ceiling or the lowest part of the roof is higher than that!

Loose boxes need to provide shelter and clean air without draughts – not always easy. A conventional outdoor box with a double-leaved door normally has its top door open all the time unless the weather is blowing directly in during colder times of year. Such a box also usually has, on the same side as the door, one window with an upper part opening inwards, which obviously needs to be higher than the horse's head to prevent him banging his head on it. The wall between a neighbouring box is often solid so the horse cannot even see his neighbours unless they all have their heads over their doors. Even then, they cannot touch and enjoy that important tactile communication and comfort. This basic

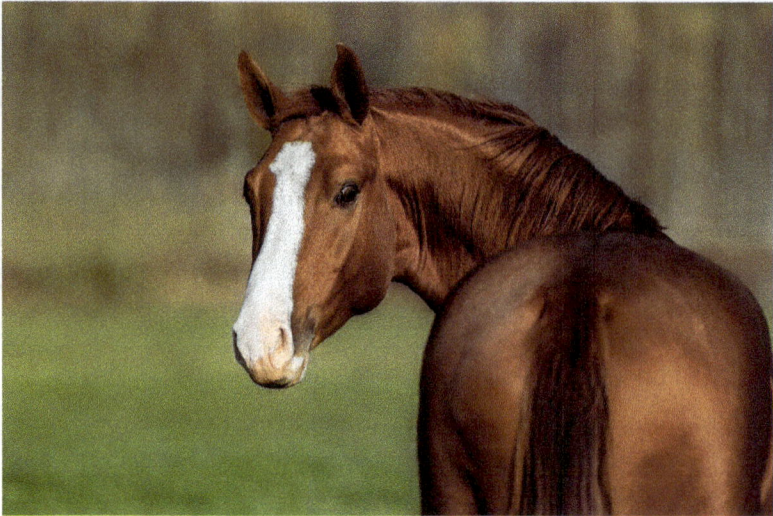

Figure 4.1 Horses are beautifully equipped to be fully aware of their surroundings during all their waking hours. This photograph shows how they can quickly see all around them with a swing of the head. When grazing, their eyes being placed high on the sides of their heads gives them an all-round view.

Their flaring nostrils can detect smells easily and permit rapid exchange of vast quantities of air should they need to gallop off to safety. Their ears can move easily, quickly and independently, from front to back to detect and identify sounds. These are all safety features needed by a prey animal.

Source: (Shutterstock ID: 2191905109)

accommodation is common but very basic and lacking in certain design features that would give its occupant much more interest and company.

Firstly, the dividing walls could be replaced by vertical railings (too close for a horse to get a hoof through) from above the double, lower wall with kicking boards; this allows some tactile contact and, of course, enables the horses to see each other more readily. There is a well-meaning school of thought which recommends that the dividing walls should be at back height with no railings or fillers above them, to allow horses to mutual groom, but there is always the chance that horses might try to get over them to join their neighbour and get stuck. There could be adjustable openings or preferably windows on the back walls, and the side walls of end boxes. Investigations could be made about modern drainage flooring to permit the drainage of urine away from the bedding. In warm or hot

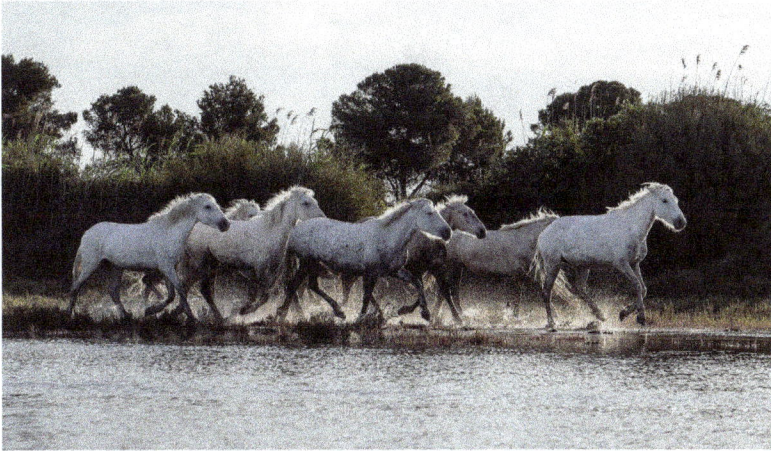

Figure 4.2 These feral horses in the French Camargue use not only all their senses to help their survival but also their strong herd instinct. Their watery environment, to which they can retreat readily, deters most predators. I have no idea if crocodiles exist in the Camargue!
Source: (Courtesy Alamy)

weather the lower doors could be fastened back and the horse kept in (with all windows opened as well) by means of a rope or strong mesh material across the space to allow air flow.

Stable fittings could be made more horse-friendly, if necessary, by making mangers and drinkers low enough for the horse to use them with his poll lower than his withers – the natural level for best ingestion of food and water: they should have rounded lower edges to protect the horse's knees. Hay holders can take the form of fixed but movable (for cleaning) large tubs on the ground, haynets at head height or holders at breast height running the length of the back wall or the half wall next to the door. Windows, of course, should be protected unless of unbreakable material like strong plastic. A valuable addition is a ridge-roof ventilator with protective cowling to allow stale air to rise up and leave the box: an open box door is a help but warm air rises and a roof ventilator would improve the horse's airspace nevertheless and, therefore, his respiratory health.

A wonderful addition, if at all possible, is to make pens behind, in front of or at the sides of boxes with openings to allow horses to come and go and give them much more of a sense of freedom. These are very popular with horses, particularly when, in reasonable weather, they can be fed outside in their pen and also communicate with their neighbours.

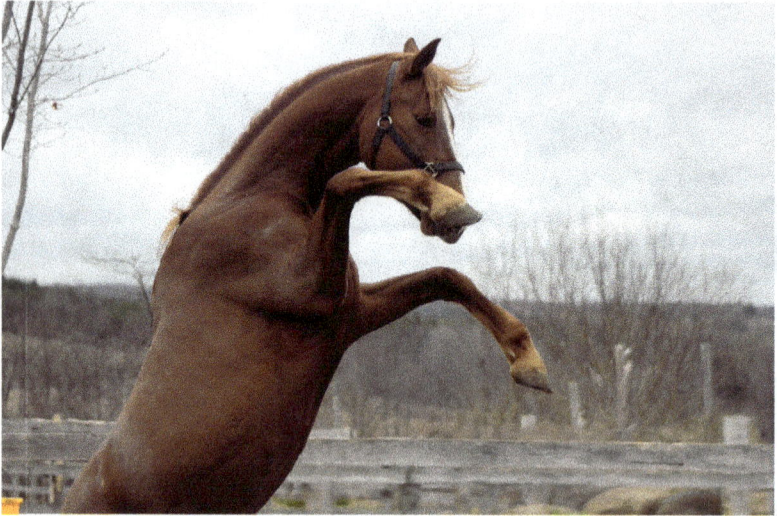

Figure 4.3 Rearing is an excellent and very impressive deterrent against adversaries or predators that have cornered a horse. A rearing horse with flailing fore hooves is a formidable animal.
Source: (Shutterstock ID: 1246952920)

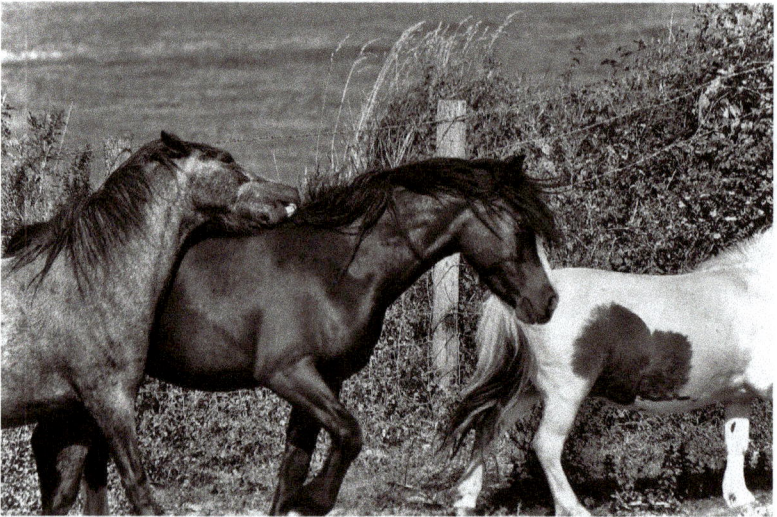

Figure 4.4 When one horse moves off with intent others often follow. Horses are curious, intelligent animals. Playing *en route* is quite acceptable.
Source: (Shutterstock ID: 2358942663)

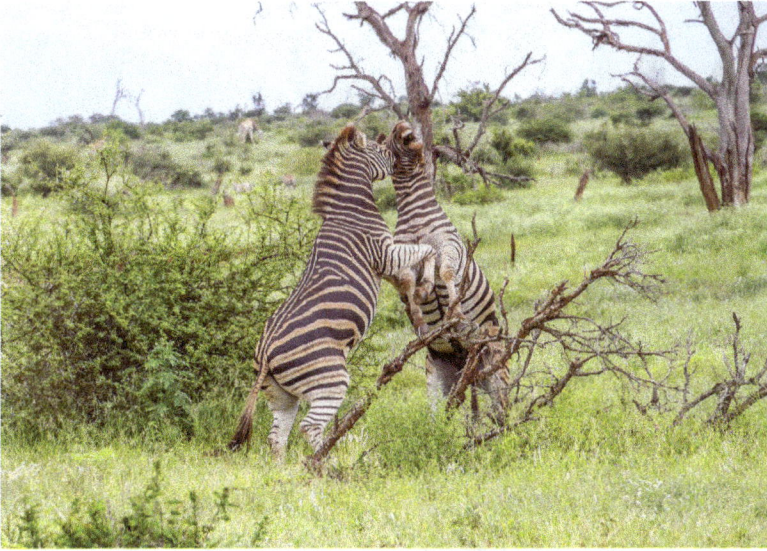

Figure 4.5 Equines of another sort. These two Burchell's zebras display equine behaviour whether playing or fighting.

Source: (Shutterstock ID: 1649650024)

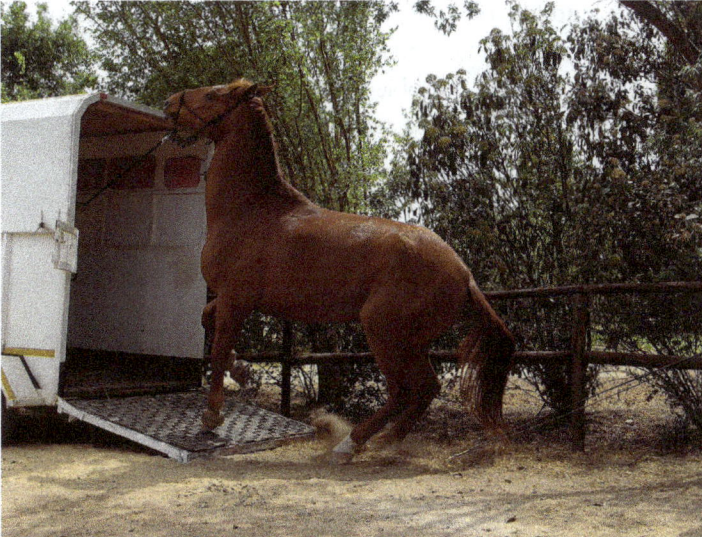

Figure 4.6 A very common sight! As prey animals, horses are very ready to object to anything seen as even slightly dangerous, like small spaces, darkness, little headroom and humans acting like predators.

Source: (Shutterstock ID: 1216418497)

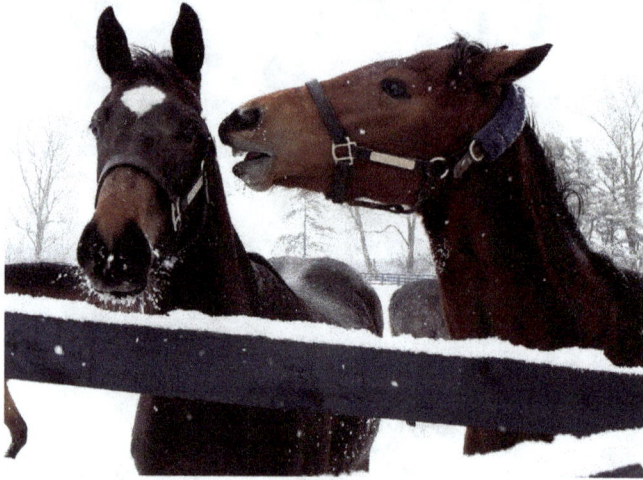

Figure 4.7 Watch out! She's going to throw a snowball!
(Shutterstock ID: 69461758)

If your establishment has a large barn (or an indoor school), this provides an excellent exercise facility for horses in adverse weather or when the natural ground is too wet for turning out. The floor surface of a barn needs to be even and not littered with anything at all, horses being inquisitive and prone to testing out objects by chewing them. Machinery or equipment of any kind needs to be securely and safely fenced off, usually in the corners, if it cannot be stored elsewhere. Surfaces in indoor schools are expensive to replace and are certainly subject to much wear and tear, but the premises *are* for the horses and they need freedom every day under normal conditions. I am not a fan of horse-walkers but admit they do provide an exercise facility if all else fails.

Paddocks and turnout areas can be made more useful and horse-friendly by the addition of shelter-sheds: in fact, these should be regarded as essential if there is no really effective natural shelter such as fairly dense tree cover. Tall, thick hedges are good but, of course, do not provide overhead shelter during rain or snow and may not protect against hot sun in summer.

Outdoor horses often need more help in the form of insect repellant, mud fever protection cream (cattle udder cream being excellent) and seasonally-appropriate rugs or sheets for use in more extreme weather conditions. Clothing of any kind needs to fit very well indeed and have frequent supervision because outdoor horses move around a lot more

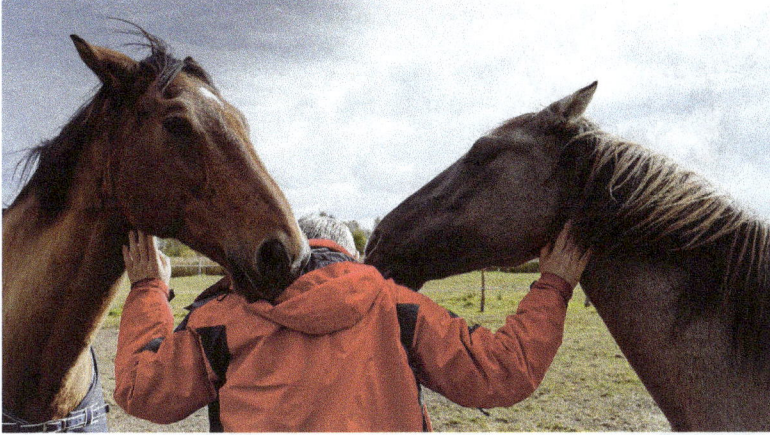

Figure 4.8 Being nuzzled to show friendship can be rather overpowering at times.
Source: (Shutterstock ID: 2137280015)

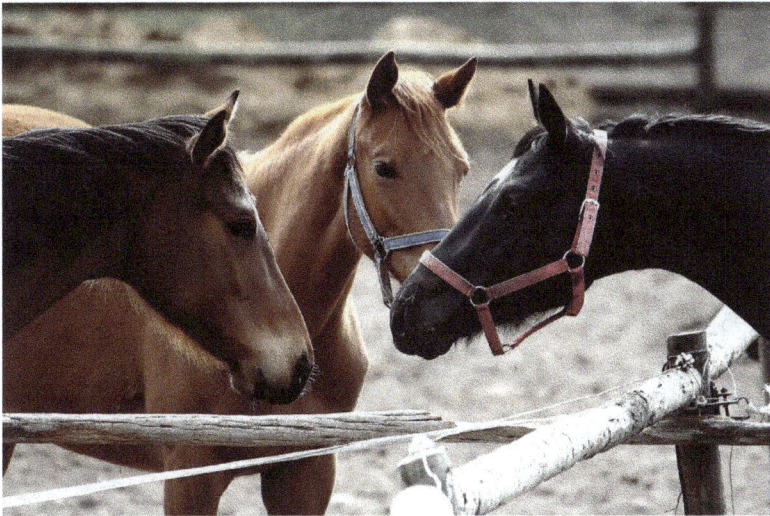

Figure 4.9 Group chat. Three horses conversing amicably.
Source: (Shutterstock ID: 5425159)

than stabled ones, get down to rest and also roll, so the rugs need to shift back into place naturally as the horses move, as, indeed, should any rug.

Water is obviously crucial to horses' health and needs checking for availability and cleanliness daily. Troughs and in-stable fittings need to

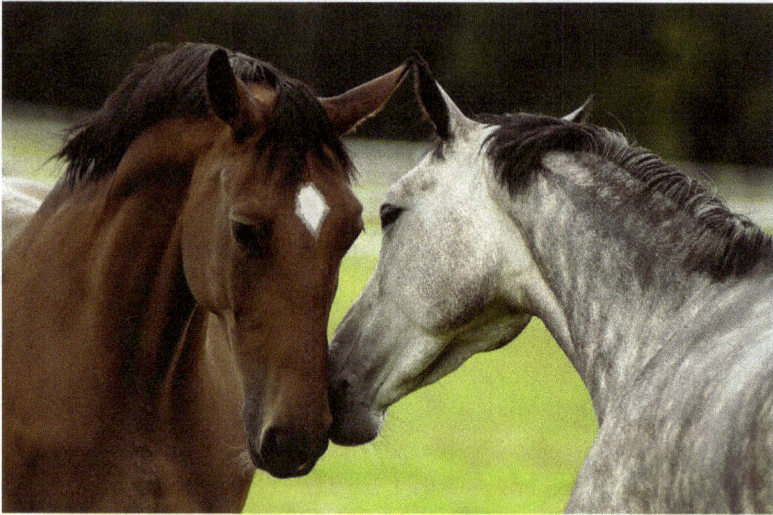

Figure 4.10 Nostril-to-nostril sniffing is a common means of friendly and exploratory communication and greeting between horses – and other species. I am sure horses feel hurt when we humans push them away when they do this with us.

Source: (Shutterstock ID: 471207410)

be safe (no sharp corners or edges). If outdoor horses rely on a stream running through their paddocks, care must be taken that they cannot wander up and down it to access areas other than their own paddocks! Also, the bottoms of streams and ponds need to be regularly checked for anything that could injure the horses – not easy. A well-managed pond, not particularly deep, is a great favourite with most horses and they often lie down in them in hot weather.

There are various types of fencing available now, mainly modelled on traditional post and rail fencing. Fencing of any kind must obviously be safe and unable to wound or even just scratch the horses in any way. The top rail of fencing, or the top band in the case of synthetic fencing, should come right to the top of the posts so that horses cannot injure themselves on their top corners, and should be slightly higher than the back of the tallest horse to use the paddock, a good deal more than this for stallions or horses prone to jumping out. The rails should be on the paddock side of the posts so that the horses do not injure their shoulders on the posts when cantering along the fence line. Of course, any fencing on which horses could injure themselves, such as barbed wire, has no place on a horse establishment, and neither does sheep netting because horses can easily get their hooves and legs through its wire squares. Ordinary wire netting is, of course, useless and potentially dangerous. Three-rail fencing is popular but four-rail is obviously more secure.

Your time and transport availabilities may influence how often you can get to see your horse if he is not on your own premises, but, as mentioned earlier, perhaps you could share your chores with a friend who has a different schedule from you, so you can help each other with your horses, perhaps with riding, or leading out to graze when turnout is restricted or just for a change. For the latter, depending on the weather, the horse should wear a rug or sheet which makes him easily visible to any traffic you may encounter if you are going off the premises. You yourself could wear a fluorescent tunic as well, plus gloves for leading and comfortable, protective boots. The horse should wear a bridle for reasonable control rather than a halter or headcollar, if going out on public roads. The best bit, I find, for grazing a horse out is a shaped, jointed snaffle with a lozenge in the middle and loose rings. These are comfortably mobile and allow the horse to move the bit around easily to manipulate the grass in his mouth and swallow it easily: grass can easily clamp up into an unchewable wad with a half-moon bit or, of course, a double bridle.

I hope some of these ideas may help you improve your horse's environment and lifestyle, whether at livery or your home, plus making life easier for you, knowing your horse is happier living in more horse-friendly facilities. I think many more horses than we realise suffer from claustrophobia, maybe only mildly, but anything we can do to create a more open feel to his stabling in particular is well worth the expense and effort. If there is trouble available, too, horses will find it so if we cultivate a safety-first mindset we can avoid most of it.

Mental State

Five

5.1 BRAIN FUNCTION IN HORSES AS OPPOSED TO HUMANS

We all know that horses are prey animals who, by nature, are 'spooky' – easily startled and not always easily settled down again. When presented with anything new, unlike some other animals such as humans, cats and dogs (all predators by nature), most equines are initially suspicious rather than curious, sometimes investigating the new object while, at the same time, partially backing off, just in case! This is a well-worn survival tactic among prey animals and is not 'silly' or cowardly. It certainly does not merit punishment of any kind. It is true that some, usually more experienced and/or older equines appear more curious and trusting, even interested, in investigating new circumstances, surroundings or objects, but many others are wary and ready to flee at any instant when faced with anything new.

This can be a make or break time for them. As herd animals, they gain great comfort, confidence and learning from others who are elder herd members, experienced at life and how to respond. They build up stock reactions to such things as predatory animals obviously targeting them, new objects or other animals in their environment and unfamiliar sounds, and learn to react accordingly in whatever is a safe way to cope with that particular perceived threat. This is why wise equestrians often train youngsters in the company of older, calm and steadying horses, and why experienced, sensible and, again that word, calm humans are best for educating youngsters.

Here is another true story. At a large college offering various equine courses up to degree level, an experiment was staged in its indoor school which had been devised by the teaching staff and never used before. It involved their building in the school a 'frightening' but static and silent pile of objects, a bit taller than a human, made up of various things from around the stables, covered by blankets, some brightly coloured items and sited several paces away from the entrance to the school so that the horses would enter but then see the pile. The point of this experiment was to

DOI: 10.1201/9781003396376-6

see how the horses of various ages would react to this 'monster', having never seen anything like it before. This was explained to the students sitting in the gallery, and they were asked which horses would kick up the most fuss at the sight of it – the youngsters or the single, older and very experienced college horse. The students were of the most common school-leaver age and just above plus a small group of mature students: all the students were experienced around horses.

It was thought by the younger students, reasonably enough, that the young horses would spook at the 'monster', but one mature student said she thought it would be the older horse. The lecturer asked why and the student said that he was used to coming into the school, having been at the college for years, and seeing jumps, dressage arenas laid out and so on, and would be absolutely phased by seeing something completely new and startling. The doors were opened and the young horses came in, loose, one by one, paying little attention to the monster, although one pawed at it until it was in danger of collapsing. Then the older horse came in and, sure enough, he 'flattened' at the sight of the pile then galloped hell for leather down to the other end of the school (not, interestingly enough, back out of the door he had just come in by) and stood, quarters in a corner, eyes on stalks and ears pricked hard, every muscle attuned to galloping off except that there was nowhere to go. A lesson on brain function in the raw.

What is the significance of my telling you this story? Horses' brains are much smaller for their size than are humans' brains, and there is another crucial difference in structure from the human brain – horses do not have what is called a pre-frontal cortex to their brains. The pre-frontal cortex, when present in other animals, is situated at the front of the brain and is responsible for many important functions, but two of the most important when we are comparing our brains with those of horses are the abilities to rationalise and analyse. This accounts for their naturally spooky nature and tendency to turn and bolt away from anything frightening. Of course, if horses did this all the time they would not be so popular as a friend and workmate so it is clear that horses *can* be accustomed, trained, to greatly modify this tendency, but we cannot insert a pre-frontal cortex into their brains. They learn by habitual, *calm*, gradual repetition to accept strange objects, surroundings, smells, sounds and so on. People who are impatient, who punish horses who do not instantly behave as they would wish, who do not understand how horses cope with the world or, even worse, who lumber them with human-like brain function, have no place among them, let alone attempting to 'train' them. Regarding horses as 'stupid' by our estimation is not only unjust and inaccurate but also counter-productive because it adversely affects how we treat them: they are not stupid, just different. Thrashing a suspicious or fleeing horse will only confirm to him that he was right to put as much distance as possible between him and 'It' – and a great deal of mental and physical harm will have been done.

It has to be said that conventional horsemanship, which does not seem to be taking on board very quickly the wondrous advantages of Equitation Science let alone keeping up with its further developments due to meticulous research, is now, to me, clearly lagging behind modern-day schooling/training, riding and management and, most importantly, a more accurate and horse-friendly way of thinking about our equine companions. It often claims to be 'classically based' – not actually 'classical', you note – but, perhaps, picking and choosing a few classical pointers here and there but, in general, being a law unto itself allowing a certain harshness and coercion to have crept in over recent decades. This, surely, could be because study at even a basic scientific level of equine brain function does not seem to take place as a topic in equestrian training and examinations. I know it can be very hard to abandon methods taught by respected instructors for generations, but now, due to meticulous scientific research, we do have much more technical knowledge of the equine brain and 'persona' than previously. I feel it is our duty to take this on board for their sakes, to savour the undoubted improvements it can make to their and our lives, and help to protect equestrianism long into the future.

At the end of this book is a marvellous book by Janet L. Jones, PhD, entitled *Horse Brain, Human Brain*. I feel confident in saying that you will never view horses in the same way again after reading it. The author, a neuroscientist, has written it in such a way that we can all understand her messages and information, to the great benefit of us, our horses and our future relationship together.

5.2 CAUSES OF SUBJECTIVE FEELINGS

We all, horses, humans and other creatures alike, have opinions of our own – subjective opinions – formed either by thinking about something and coming to our own conclusion or actually experiencing it. Many of us have experience of horses who also have strongly held subjective feelings due to something that has happened to them. A client of mine had a horse who had started to be reluctant to be led into his loose box and she asked me, at the end of our lesson, if I could help to rectify this 'fault' in his behaviour. The horse looked to me as though he was worried and slightly scared of going into his box with his owner (who was not at all rough or cruel with him) so I suggested that, just outside his box, she should throw the reins, which were over his head as for leading in hand, over his withers and let him go in on his own, that is, without being led.

She was worried that, as he appeared to not want to go into his box, he would refuse and become loose on the yard but I told her I didn't think he would. She looked after him well and there was nearly always hay available in his box, plus water and bedding, and he had plenty of turnout time with his friends, so there was no obvious reason for him to be reluctant to go in, especially after being without food for some time, having had his lesson. At the entrance to his box, she halted him, draped the reins over his withers and stepped back, saying 'walk on' to him – and he walked straight in without either hesitating or rushing, waiting inside to be untacked. It then transpired, after a few queries from me, that a few days earlier the horse had accidentally bumped his owner against the door jamb when going in with his owner and had subsequently developed this new problem. He was obviously reluctant to repeat the experience and tried to show her that. The new way of entering his stable was a great success and the problem was solved.

It does normally take an experience of some kind, good or bad, for horses, and us, to form subjective opinions about anything. Horses become 'sour' in their work or daily life processes usually because it has become hard for them, frightening, painful or just unpleasant in some way. It is true that horses can develop what appear to be permanent memories of occasions, objects, people and other animals, and also retain the feelings they formed about them. If those feelings are good, fine, but if they are not the horse can demonstrate his or her dislike if a similar situation arises later in life and cause 'problems' which may not be easy to eradicate. They seem to be able to remember everywhere they have been even if it was only once years before. They remember people for better or worse and act according to how they made them feel, even from years earlier.

It is clear that everything we do with horses can create a firmly held memory about which a horse can form a subjective opinion. They can remember routes, people, incidents and situations from many years earlier so we have to be as careful as we can to avoid any negative experiences for them. Most of us buy horses who have had a life before we bought them, and their previous lives can cause perplexing problems for us unless we can work out why a horse seems worried or angry about something (and try to improve matters) or is doing something a former person in his life has trained him to do but which we don't want. Sometimes we can train him to react to these memories differently or not at all, but often we cannot and must simply try to avoid similar circumstances occurring or avoid certain situations. There is no point, in a case like this, in trying to force a horse to do things our way: our best chance is to ameliorate the occasion as best we can, which often succeeds.

So, subjective feelings can arise in a horse's mind as easily as they can in ours. We cannot get rid of them but simply may have to adapt to trying, without force, to give the horse better memories and, therefore, feelings, about similar situations in his present life, or avoiding them if we can.

5.3 THE EFFECTS OF EXPERIENCES

Similarly to the preceding section, memories of real, live experiences can live on in a horse's brain for the rest of his life. Being the type of animal they are, prey animals with brains capable of holding lifelong memories, we may not be able to re-train a horse to forget or not react to those memories but we can usually make certain that, whatever the horse is trying to show us with 'difficult' behaviour, we remember for our part that it has a cause and meant a lot, good or bad, to the horse at that time and he has every reason to expect that whatever it was might happen again.

For instance, once a horse is 'bad in traffic' he will probably never become reliably well-behaved and safe in traffic. It might just be, for example, one particular type of vehicle, one kind of noise, one particular colour, one particular location, or any of several other triggers but it may well be indelibly impressed on his brain and, even in the company of other horses immune to it, he may not be able to overcome his fear. As an example, I once knew a horse who was afraid of lorries but exactly why we were never able to find out. He was taken out with four other horses to protect him, one each side of him, one in front and one behind. He did eventually, after many months and with a sensitive, highly competent rider, greatly improve, but never to the extent of being able to be hacked out alone in case a lorry appeared on the scene.

On the brighter side, it is far from unusual, for example, for horses who have been involved in travelling accidents, such as horseboxes turning over and similar nightmares, to load perfectly into a box the very next time they are presented with this circumstance, as though the previous accident had never happened. No one, that I know of, has ever been able to explain this phenomenon. Surely there can be nothing more terrifying than to be involved in such an accident, for human or horse, yet many such horses do seem to be unaffected by the terror they must have felt. I am not the only person who has no answer to that.

5.4 CAUSES OF PAIN AND DISCOMFORT AND HOW TO ALLEVIATE THEM

The first time I was ever told to whip a horse as a punishment was when I was in my teens. My original riding teacher had retired and his school bought by another very experienced person who, however, was of a different school of thought and treated horses like the Victorians treated naughty children – harshly, to teach them a lesson. This way of thinking, of course, was and still is very common. It is prevalent among people who believe that horses think like humans and will be able to connect the pain of a beating with the way they are behaving (although they are trying to communicate with us) and, so, not behave like that again or they will be beaten. It can be very difficult, of course, to change the mind of someone who has thought in a particular way for possibly decades, no matter how patiently and clearly matters are explained to them, but, with the progress of Equitation Science and the knowledge that what is termed our Social Licence to Operate is put in clear and present danger by such behaviour, I hope that a new generation of horse people will arise to whom rationality and continuing education rather than cruelty and stubbornness are the rule. Causing pain to any creature who is trying to communicate difficulty to us or is trying to defend himself can never be acceptable.

5.5 EQUINE EMOTIONAL EXPRESSION

Covered largely in Part 3 on Health, the way a sensitive creature such as a horse expresses his emotions is a subject we really must do our best to master, not only for the sake of his well-being but also that of our own safety. Horse language is largely physical although the noises horses make are varied and expressive, and can tell us a lot.

Horse sounds are several and not limited to the familiar whinny or neigh of a horse calling out to, say, a distant friend (horse or human) as he canters over to greet them. A loud, even nearly screaming whinny indicates alarm or that the horse is trying to get someone's attention – again, horse or human; this can also mean anger, stallions being said to 'roar' at rivals. There is also the soft 'whickering' sound – a low-pitched vibrating noise – given when we are with a horse and which we take to mean affection or expectation of a treat. Then there is the squeal of sudden pain, alarm, dissention (disagreement or 'telling off') or even high excitement in play. If a horse is in sustained pain he will often make a low, moaning noise which is unmistakable and heart-wrenching.

Basically, the attitude of a horse's body, particularly his head, comprising as it does his ears and face, can tell an experienced, observant and caring horse person very clearly how he is feeling. You don't have to be an expert as such to tell if a horse is tired, not well, interested, calm, friendly, angry or any of many other emotions. It seems, very often, to be instinctive in us as fellow mammals, but, because of horses' immense strength, we need to learn as much as we can to avoid, for example, the serious injuries that can occur if we confuse interest and/or friendliness with anger and a warming to back off.

An interested horse will point his ears towards whatever is catching his attention, his eyes will be bright and well open, his nostrils may be circular and quivering as he tries to take in the smell of whatever it is and his tail may well be slightly raised. Anger, though, can be frightening in a horse. His ears will be back, his eyes unmistakably angry, his nostrils pulled up and back and his lips may be parted showing his teeth. His tail may be thrashing. He is giving us fair warning to get out of his space.

As we are responsible and being on the spot regularly with our horse, we also need to be very familiar with the look of a healthy, happy horse as opposed to one in pain, below par or sick. Individuals, in any species, can differ, of course, but the basic signs of the main emotions are important for us to learn for the mentioned reasons. A healthy, happy horse will usually have bright eyes and coat, he will have an engaged expression on his face and be paying attention to his surroundings with ears pointing towards his object of interest. His tail will probably be loose and relaxed, and he will present a picture of all being right with his world. Conversely, a sick horse feeling poorly may have dull, 'sunken' eyes, show little interest in his surroundings and ears perhaps flopping to the sides with his head held rather low. His tail (the boney part of his tail, the dock from which the hair grows and which is a continuation of his spine, of course) will be down but not stiff. A horse in pain may be moving around somewhat depending on the cause of the pain, maybe rocking from foot to foot or 'resting' a painful foot, that is, not weight-bearing on the ground. He may be moaning, getting up and down a good deal, rolling, or rocking on his feet with his head probably low, and could be moaning. His tail may be still, flicking or thrashing depending on what is wrong with him.

Any horse not showing normal behaviour needs watching closely, ideally overnight as well, as any delay, as with other animals or humans, can have serious consequences. If you are worried or uncertain, maybe due to lack of experience, it is always worth a call to your veterinary surgeon. Many people advise waiting to see if the horse improves but I do not agree with this: it is very well worth a phone call to your vet or some professional at his surgery if you are unsure, otherwise you may regret it in the future.

5.6 CALMNESS – HORSES' NATURAL STATE

If you watch a group of horses, either a feral herd or a domestic group, and stay with it for some time, you will gather that they are naturally fairly peaceful animals. As vegetarian prey animals they do not go off on expeditions looking for food (other animals to hunt down and kill) but spend most hours of their day with heads down grazing whatever they can find, and normally stay in their group together. They do travel (very roughly about 25 miles a day) to find fresh grazing, browsing and water but usually at a middling pace depending on whether their herd contains youngsters or elderly members.

(The fastest recorded speed of a galloping Thoroughbred racehorse is 43.97 mph, while the top speed of a hunting cheetah in a short burst is 70 mph. Compare this with rather slower wild or feral equidae and remember that the Thoroughbred record was taken on a ridden horse, also that cheetahs do not often hunt zebras, for example, but find smaller, lighter animals easier to catch, and you will understand why equines survived so long as truly wild animals, only becoming strictly speaking extinct as wild horses as opposed to feral ones due to human interference. Formerly wild horses today (such as the Przewalski) which are being reintroduced to their original homelands are correctly referred to now as feral even if they were born in the wild. The top speed of, say, a lion hunting zebra will be up to about 37 mph in short bursts, and of a zebra around the same. Please forgive this diversion which, I hope, is nevertheless interesting.)

The one emotion established herds of feral horses show most of is calmness. Grazing and browsing have a definite soporific effect on equines. This is what they evolved for and were born to do. They exude peacefulness, contentment and happiness when they are quietly eating what nature provides for them. Their structure of four fairly thin legs, long necks and heads with eyes placed high up on the sides of their heads is ideal for keeping an eye out for hunting predators while continuing to take in grasses, leaves from trees and shrubbery and other vegetation. Having said that, it has to be said also that horses can be what we might call nervous – they react like lightning to anything that startles them and, if free, will take off and get to a safe distance (unless being pursued) without thinking about it. Remember the lack of logic and reason due to their lack of a pre-frontal cortex. This makes their motto, if they have one, 'run first, think later' as many of us may know to our cost!

Generally 'messing around with horses' in the stable yard often involves their being tethered to a ring or something else strongly fixed, either in the stable or on the yard and, to a horse, this is a most dangerous situation. Youngsters have to be gradually trained to be restricted in this way. Fear takes over horses almost instantaneously and even the best rider can find themselves run away with for several or many yards/metres before regaining control. To keep sensitive and potentially nervous animals like horses in an appropriate way for them and a safe one for us involves the need to keep them as calm as possible as much as possible. A solitary existence, even for a short while in the field or yard when all others are not nearby, can put almost any horse on edge even if they do not always give out physical signs to inform us. We do require horses to work alone quite often, including hacking, but they do need to be accustomed to this and to the knowledge that, when they return, there will be other horses around.

In their own down time, horses do much better, on the whole, if they can not only see others but touch them, mutual groom with them, socialise with them, play with them if so inclined and generally be horses together. When turned out, friendships must be considered and new horses on a yard gradually introduced, in hand, to another mild-natured one to welcome them and show them the ropes. More and more stabling today is being constructed, if new, or altered to provide not merely 'chat holes' in dividing walls but vertical railings so that the horses can see all around and take in the presence of others. This kind of life when stabled is very much more horse-friendly when you have compatible neighbours and promotes contentment, which is so important to horses.

5.7 BOREDOM

A horse's 'natural' life, even in a domestic field, does not, clearly, involve him or her becoming bored because there is always company, food and, hopefully, clean water available. Boredom is not a natural state for horses, but countless numbers of them certainly do experience it when confined, whether in stables or, if alone, on a small yard leading to their box or used to 'exercise' horses when not ridden. In this situation, boredom can be the cause of the horses trying to jump out and perhaps sustaining injuries in their search for other equine company.

Horses who are exercised daily by being turned loose with others (of compatible temperaments) or by being ridden, led out or exercised loose do not suffer from boredom to anything like the same extent as their more confined yard-mates, but one hour a day out of their stables is very poor relief from the confinement otherwise suffered. More and more, caring horse people are making efforts to see that their horses are out with others as much as is reasonably possible, allowing for weather, appropriate company and all the other conditions that make life worth living for horses. This can be very difficult on, for instance, livery yards run on strict, old-fashioned lines, but, for the well-being and, yes, the health and welfare of the horses, it is now accepted that facilities need to be improved. Attitudes towards horses' needs also call for improvement in cases where horses are over-restricted, and such yards and practices can only be regarded, in this day and age, as not fit for their purpose of housing horses and promoting their well-being.

There are such things as horse toys marketed mainly in horse magazines and these can provide some light relief for the horses. They are only short-term solutions on any particular day, though, and a horse's main source of occupation is not only eating appropriate food but being able to socialise with friends. I have always found that an effective way of easing boredom for horses if grazing and/or equine company are restricted is leading them out in hand, singly or with a friend, to graze on carefully chosen areas, ideally away from traffic. This gives them a welcome change of not only scenery but also tasty food of a different flavour from that normally available. If paddocks are not managed well, the grass in them becomes sour, perhaps infested with equine parasites if droppings are not regularly picked up (not scattered by harrowing which makes things worse), and a trip out to eat grass growing freely outside paddocks is a very welcome relief that horses really enjoy. It is even better if a friend can accompany you on your trip out. Even half an hour is better than nothing.

5.8 FRUSTRATION

I believe that many more horses than is realised experience frustration with their lives and work. Horses are hard-wired to their natural way of life no matter how long the species has been domesticated and I think that modern riding in general contributes to frustration because of its harshness compared with techniques and attitudes that prevailed a few decades ago. Of course, there has always been the attitude that a horse is an animal and, therefore, inferior to human beings but, even if some people believe that, it does not mean that it is in order to gratuitously treat them in ways that upset them such as over-confinement or giving them insufficient roughage feed, or riding techniques that cause them to move in ways contrary to their physique and natural action because that way of going is popular in their particular competitive discipline. There is also the fact that many working horses do not have enough freedom or opportunity to socialise normally with other horses for fear of their being injured. There is actually very little risk of this if only horses friendly towards each other are turned loose together.

A very obvious practice that contributes to frustration is the strong, modern bit contact now often used and the tight bridles and, especially, nosebands inflicted on many horses. The standard rule of bridle and bit fit – that of being able to slide a finger *easily* under all straps on the horse's head including the noseband where two fingers' width actually is recommended between the straps around the jaws and the horse's head – and that bits should not be hoisted up so high that more than one wrinkle is created at the corners of a horse's mouth – should always be obeyed for the horse's welfare. Saddles and girths can cause problems, as mentioned earlier, because saddles are so often put on too far forward so that the tops of the horse's shoulder blades are bruised, and the girth also is pulled forward and bruises the horse behind the elbows. The girth, of course, should be tightened just enough to keep the saddle securely in place, not hoisted up so tight that you cannot get the top halves of your fingers between it and the horse's ribs.

What do these basic fitting parameters, and a horse's way of going, have to do with a horse's frustration? Simply that both can cause considerable discomfort, restriction and even pain. The horse is trying to move as required but any of the aforementioned three will frustrate (!) his ability and willingness to do so, which usually results in increased pressure, even force in some cases, from his rider. And what about the modern way of going that most riders seem to adopt? Again, we all know the expert advice that a horse's poll should be the highest point of his outline (ears not counted) and the flat bone down the front of his face, the nasal planum, should be at most vertical to the ground from forehead to muzzle and ideally just in front of the vertical. In addition to low polls with the highest point of the horse's outline being about a third of the way down the crest of his neck, and the front of his face BTV – behind the vertical – we can see that many horses' necks look shorter than natural because the rider is actually pulling the head in quite forcefully, causing all three of these faults. Secondary results from this are a weakened, dropped back instead of the stronger, protective, slightly lifted back, plus insufficient forward tracking and weight-bearing of the hind legs. These defensive postures of the horse can cause him not only pain but also injuries. As this book is not specifically about training, I recommend that readers consult my book *Fine Riding* for the remedy for these faults plus a stronger body and happier mind for the horse.

Other frustrating situations for horses are not being able to spend enough time with equine friends although probably being able to see, hear and smell them, insufficient roughage food (hay, haylage), insufficient freedom with friendly company and too much confinement, feed containers which may be difficult to eat out of such as small buckets or too lightweight so they are unstable, any container sited too high, haynets with tiny holes, friends turned out in a different field from them, uncomfortable clothing that he can do nothing about – you get the picture. What bothers one horse may not worry another, so, as ever, it is up to those who care for and work the horse most (a) to recognise and correct what is inappropriate for him in his lifestyle, and (b) find out by studying him what he likes, what makes him happy and settled, and go all out to provide it for him.

5.9 HAPPINESS

So far as I know, there is still no official acceptance of horses experiencing happiness. The British government only about a couple of years ago, at the time of writing this book, announced that it was now recognised that animals are sentient, so expecting some formal declaration that animals can be happy is perhaps expecting a bit too much. Those of us who have a real feel for our animals, who study them formally and/or informally to uncover what makes each individual happy and go out of our way to bring these captive, domestic animals joy, indeed, happiness, can just carry on looking for happiness in our animals and doing what we can to establish it firmly and securely in each and every one of them. Personally, I find it a tremendous compliment when an animal of any species makes it unarguably plain that he or she is pleased to see you when you turn up at the yard or come home after time away. I love the way they take charge of and fit into the environment you have provided for them, often at the expense of your own comfort, the way they happily follow the, in this case, horse-friendly routine and practices you have instilled and generally meld into your life, and you into theirs. This is a true partnership strengthened by mutual affection – in some humans' cases, sheer besottedness!

But what can you do if you know that your horse is not happy, even just not as happy as he could be? Most owners who have their own place are usually in a position to alter facilities and maybe also their own timetable and practices to fit in better with their horse's needs: it is when we are keeping horses on someone else's place that problems can develop, and it is surprising how conditions can change once your horse is installed. Most responsible, reputable livery yard owners offer, and expect to exchange, signed contracts detailing conditions, prices, what you can and cannot do and what they will and won't do for their part of the bargain. But I find there is usually a clause over-riding all these conditions at the wish of the yard owner, which they claim is necessary to cover unforeseen circumstances. This may be understandable from their point of view, but it can make life very difficult for their clients and their horses if changes make life and conditions worse for you and/or your horse. You may have no choice but to leave which, in itself, can make things even worse if it means your horse has to leave his best friend or friends, or you are faced with a longer trip to see and 'do' him, or things turn out to be not what you expected.

I have been through all this and sympathise with those who are landed with unwanted circumstances while congratulating those who have found another Happy Place for themselves and their horse or horses. The really important points are, will you be happy if your horse is not and if he or she is happy, are you able to absorb any inconveniences or expenses to keep it that way?

5.10 SADNESS

I was once at a large yard teaching some of the clients when, during a chat with them in a stable block after the lessons, I suddenly felt a wave of great sadness from behind me. I turned and saw a horse (not one I had been teaching) with his head over his door looking very unhappy. I went over to him and he pushed his head into my chest and rocked slightly. I cuddled and stroked him for a minute, then asked the clients whose horse he was and why he was so sad. One woman told me matter-of-factly that he was one of her horses and he was missing his friend who had been sold off the yard a few days earlier. I suggested a few things to make him happier, but she said she couldn't do all that and he would just have to get used to it. I must say she didn't seem to care about it at all.

Many people do not realise just how sensitive and emotional horses are, most animals, in fact, and that they suffer from loss, change, confusing treatment, pain and other negative circumstances, just as we do. My heart went out to him not just because he had lost his closest friend with, of course, no understanding of why, but also because his owner did not care about his sadness at all and was not even prepared to try to help him.

Sadness does seem to not be considered by many horse people. When substantial changes occur in their horses' lives they just seem to think that the horse will get used to or over it in a couple of days or a week and that will be that. However, I do know that horses' sadness and also the confusion and worry of changing homes and companions can last for several weeks and result in poor appetite, apparent lack of energy and interest in anything, and even the development of stereotypical behaviours (see later). While changes may be impossible to prevent, we can, even though we are not fellow equines, help a little by spending more time with our horse, sensing whether he would like a gentle massage or some other comforting attention but definitely not be chivvied along cheerfully, made to work and so on, as though that would make him feel better, which it almost certainly would not. Being turned out with others might help, but I have found that leading such a horse out to graze does seem to take his mind off his predicament somewhat. He has different grass to choose from and the company of a human he likes and trusts. Ultimately, trying to find him another equine friend, if possible, really helps – and the stable cats can also play a valuable role here, many of whom seem to love dozing on horses backs!

5.11 ANXIETY

I am sure that this emotion is far more common in horses than we realise. If we think about what we already know, horses have very little real control over their lives. We cannot explain to them what is going to happen in the near future, that their neighbour will be back in an hour or so, that the vet will do his or her best not to hurt them and so on. Calming a horse with a soothing voice using long-drawn-out sounds can certainly help and stroking fairly firmly and slowly is also very reassuring. Patting should always be avoided because it feels just like the short, sharp shock feeling of being kicked or bitten by another horse and does not have the right effect at all. Stroking, or rubbing much like horses mutually grooming or massaging each other with their front teeth, can certainly calm them down and relax them. I often wonder why those competitors who slap and thump their horses hard after doing well, usually in a competition, do not think about how awful such a sensation feels to their poor horses.

I was trained by the late Pamela Hannay as an equine shiatsu therapist, which is a therapy between acupuncture (using no needles) and massage – a kind of acupressure – and have always found it wonderful for really relaxing horses. I gave sessions to retired racehorses at a specialist yard for some time, where one of the grooms was interested in the technique. She told me, after I had treated a particularly difficult box-walker one day, that for a whole hour after my departure the mare did not box walk at all but stood, head down dozing, which was very unusual: she was normally on the move most of the time.

That mare was in a permanently anxious state, but most of our horses only display anxiety, which can be very subtle, occasionally or in certain situations. Gentle, confident treatment from us can help them greatly plus trying to 'water down' or prevent whatever is causing the anxiety. Perhaps unexpectedly and all other factors considered, I find it often helps horses prone to anxiety to be stabled and turned out with very confident and/or quiet horses as their nonchalance seems to rub off.

5.12 FEAR

This is one emotion that most horse owners are very familiar with in their horses. Horses, as prey animals, are quick to become alarmed by, in domesticity, almost anything unfamiliar, noisy, smelly or that looks really weird – to them. It is also a highly dangerous emotion for them and particularly for us weakling humans because horses react to fear without thinking, due to their lack of a pre-frontal cortex in their brains, explained earlier, and can easily flatten us with catastrophic effects. They can run through wooden fencing, crash into trees or buildings, cars and anything else that is in their direct path away from danger.

As a boy early last century, my father witnessed a frightful incident concerning a horse and cart (common then) outside his home. The driver had stopped in the street to deliver something to a house when a loud noise from well behind the horse frightened him and he set off, totally panic-stricken, at a fast gallop, obviously cart and all, down the street, people flying out of the way terrified. At the end of the street the horse could have turned left or right because straight in front of him was a brick wall but, in his sheer panic, when horses do not think but are taken over by their survival instincts, the horse galloped at full speed into the wall, killing himself instantly. It shocked everybody and my father never forgot it. Nevertheless, he let me start riding lessons at 4 years of age.

On the best-run horse establishments, great emphasis is laid on employing calm, strong-minded, knowledgeable and caring employees (which I am told are getting harder and harder to find!) because they exude just the required atmosphere to create a secure haven for horses. Noisy people who rush about, scream, laugh loudly and shout or clang buckets, drop things on the ground or hassle the horses are the very worst kind of staff. At a minimum, they disturb the horses' natural equanimity and bring to the surface irritation and the wariness that can lead to more violent emotions in the equine brain, which are not difficult to trigger. They can also put these captive, sensitive and far-from-stupid animals off their feed and even, in extremes, trigger 'stable vices' (see later). No running except in real emergencies and no loud noises should be the order of the day, every day.

What about radios? At Ireland's National Stud, when innovative veterinary surgeon Michael Osborne was in charge, they ran some research experiments on general horse topics, one of which was the effects on horses of music. They found that horses seemed to like radios playing certain music but only for up to 30 minutes at a time (and not very often), after which the horses showed signs of irritation and restlessness, head nodding, teeth grinding, swaying and so on. The types of music they liked were quiet, and included military music, much tuneful classical music and gentle background music. They seemed to like ballads, but, for the most part, they disliked the sound of the human voice! That's us told.

5.13 ANTICIPATION

Horses, of course, get used to well-maintained daily routines and living on a well-ordered yard, and slot into the timetable readily provided if it is horse-friendly and they know they will have whatever they need most of the time – hay, feed, turnout, company if not as close as they would like, exercise, a comfortable, clean bed, grooming and so on. This can be a double-edged sword because they anticipate these events throughout the day and can become worried or anxious if they don't happen when expected. Horses also, I am certain, dread being ridden or worked by certain people and do their best for others. Modern ideas and techniques of riding and training create much happier and healthier horses.

I have found for a couple of decades that the combination of true classical riding plus the application of modern Equitation Science techniques is certainly the way to go and well worth researching if you are not familiar with them.

One of my professional visits was to a large police stables, obviously to write about the horses' intriguing training, their use and management principles. In those days, most such horses were kept tethered in stalls, with a few 'special cases' in loose boxes, and their work meant that they were taken out and brought home at very varying times of day and evening, and occasionally at night, so there was no routine as such. I queried the effects of this with the officer in charge, who told me that because there was always hay and water available waiting for them when they came in, whatever time it was, the horses did not become upset at the constant comings and goings and the not knowing when or whether they would be going out. There were grass turn-out facilities at the yard, but the horses were turned out singly to avoid accidents. (I can understand this logic but have always found that accidents are virtually non-existent if only friendly horses are turned out together, and they enjoy their turnout time much more, to their mental benefit, if they have the company of a friend.)

The police horses were rarely without human attention and seemed well-routined, although I did notice that many of them readily kicked and bit people! I queried this, as well, and the officer explained it away by saying that they were used to high-tension occasions (if not as a matter of course) and horses were highly-strung, anyway. Hmm. Not exactly a reason for biting and kicking. During my day there, I took in the stable practices and the horses' circumstances when in their stalls.

It did not seem to make any difference to their behaviour whether they were in loose boxes or stalls. The officer in charge told me proudly that the stables had been especially architect-designed to provide only the best surroundings for the horses. Unfortunately, the architect clearly had not known anything about horses or, apparently, asked those involved in the nitty-gritty of horse hands-on care. He had, though, consulted several horse books on how to accommodate and look after horses.

The first things I noticed were the hay racks higher than the horses' heads – 'for safety' – making it certain that bits of hay would fall into the horses' eyes. The tie rings, through which the headcollar ropes passed, at breast height, with wooden weights on the ends, seemed alright but the arrangement for short feeds was amazing. This consisted of wells set down into the floor of each stable so that the level of the feed would gradually sink lower and lower below ground level as the horse ate, meaning that, in theory, he could only clean up if he bent his knees and crouched down to finish his feed – impossible for a horse – or splayed his forelegs uncomfortably sideways or one in front and one behind like a young foal, so he could get his head down to his feed! I was told that the architect had proudly explained that the books all said that horses should eat from ground level (so what about the hay which they spend most time eating?) and so he had innovatively designed these special 'mangers'. The officer in charge also told me that, for some reason, almost none of the horses did, in practice, eat all their feed and many were prone to pawing hard on the ground around the mangers (including those in loose boxes), prematurely wearing out the toes of their shoes and even, some of them, developing concussion lameness, so being regularly out of use.

When I explained why all this was happening and how to rectify it (lower the hayracks, fill in the wells and install static, easy-clean mangers at a height allowing the horses to eat with their polls just lower than their withers) the officer looked at me amazed and did not speak for some time, eventually emitting a naughty word followed by 'I hadn't thought of that'. Neither had anyone else, it seems. After all, as I was told, they were police officers first and horsemen and women second. Whether anything was done to rectify matters I do not know.

Of course, the tension and the frustration of knowing there was feed there all the time that they could not reach must have been awful for the horses and could have gone some way towards explaining why so many were ill-at-ease to the extent that they readily bit and kicked. Poor things.

So far as our current topic, anticipation, is concerned, a well-timed, horse-friendly routine is essential for settled, happy and thriving horses. This does not mean that changes cannot be made and confident (see next) horses will adapt fairly easily, but, in general, they need to know where they stand, confident that they will have all their needs attended to and roughly when, be treated fairly and correctly and, on the whole, be happy and, therefore, healthy and content.

5.14 CONFIDENCE

Confidence! Something we all want and respect in others. The lives we make horses lead do not, on the whole, promote confidence in them. The equestrian industry, apparently worldwide, does not seem to have any effective regulation as to its conduct and its treatment of the horses on which it depends. Horses can be bred and bought by anyone from almost anywhere and some, indeed many, horses and ponies, not to mention donkeys, seem to be in the hands of people far from ethically qualified to be in charge of their well-being. We do not even have, at least in the UK where I live, an official, government-run licence scheme to formally inform 'the authorities' that we own, are responsible for and capable of looking after a horse.

What creates or destroys confidence in horses? Confidence is the main aspect of a horse's life that makes him feel safe – confidence that the humans who are looking after and working with them will not hurt or frighten them. If a horse is caused pain or fear, or even discomfort, even once, in any aspect of his life that he connects with humans, that knocks his confidence in us, and horses have tremendously long memories. This places us in a risky position because, of course, horses are prey animals and any kind of danger encourages them to run away from it. Once a horse has been hurt in a particular situation he will be on his guard if that set of circumstances occurs again because he is made that way, he has that mindset, and guarding himself against a similar situation soon becomes a hard-wired part of his personal survival kit. We can use our voices to soothe him and he will recognise a calming tone, but we can't promise him that whatever it was that frightened or hurt him won't happen again.

All this means that we need to learn and put into practice everything we reasonably can about horses and I am afraid it also means that we can never fully relax in their company, either on the ground, riding or driving. We can have 'full confidence' in our horses and they can trust us as well, but some things occur for which neither of us can plan. In these cases, the stronger our bond and the more our horse trusts us, which he learns from our behaviour and his lifestyle, then the more likely it is that we'll weather whatever storm has currently struck us, that he will probably calm down when we tell him to, so that, generally, he feels that he is safe with us. This demands knowledge and self-control from us.

If we have ever had the luck to come across a horseman or woman who clearly has the knack of not only thinking like a horse but of somehow transmitting that reassurance and confidence to the equines he or she deals with, we should take note of how they also make us feel as well, what they do with horses, how they move around them, how their vocal tone changes according to what they want a horse to do and note how quiet, smooth and, yes, confident in themselves they are. All this is quickly

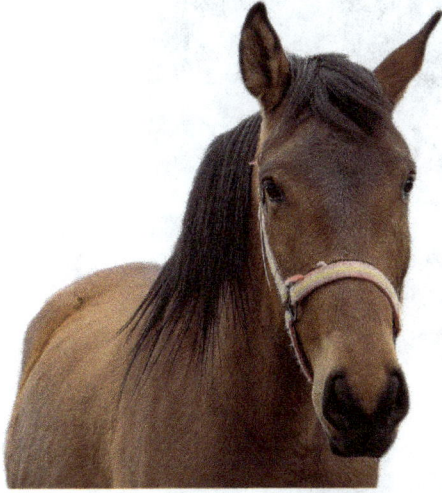

Figure 5.1 Horses are naturally herd animals, needing company in order to feel safe and settled. Most isolated horses, like this one, do not thrive very well. This horse's 'flat' appearance tells us he is not feeling happy and is maybe even feeling rather insecure.
Source: (Shutterstock ID: 303438857)

taken in by horses and they not only usually relax for such people, they co-operate with them and work with them because they feel safe. That should always be our aim.

5.15 HORSES' ENVIRONMENTAL TEMPERATURE TOLERANCES

Horses and ponies can readily tolerate temperatures lower than we can unless there is a strong wind or precipitation (sleet, snow or rain). Although in nature they are not animals who make dens or homes of any kind, they do certainly seek shelter from extremes of temperature either way, or from any unpleasant weather conditions. Their coats grow seasonally so that they are shorter in summer and longer in winter. Horses and ponies protect themselves somewhat by standing with their tails towards inclement weather. Their tails, particularly when left full on the dock, offer good protection to the thin skin between the buttocks; also, the longer hair blocks some of the wind and weather blowing through their hindlegs to the thinner skin between the legs and on their bellies. Those with longer manes not infrequently can be seen to graze with their manes towards any unfavourable weather blowing in, as body heat is lost readily from the neck.

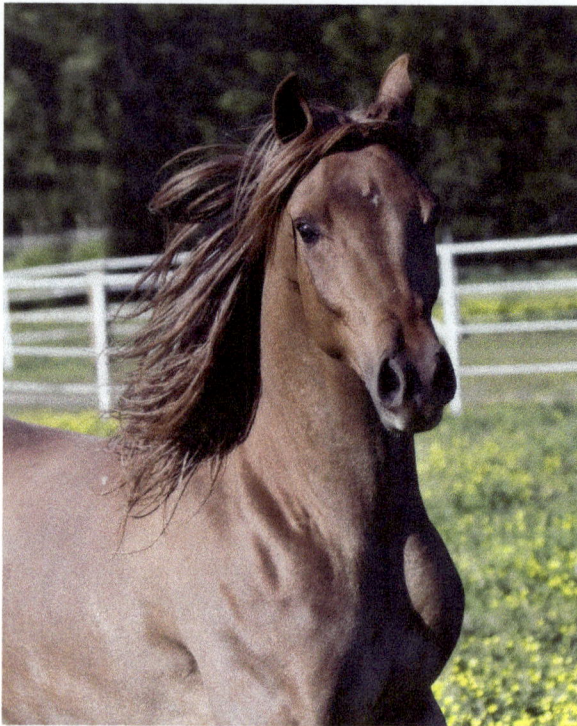

Figure 5.2 This head shot of a horse galloping free shows anxiety rather than pleasurable excitement. One ear is cocked back, perhaps towards something frightening that started the flight in the first place, and the other is directed towards the photographer. The horse's wide nostrils and tense carriage show a level of fear rather than enjoyable freedom.
Source: (Shutterstock ID: 30299464)

As with us, it is easier to protect a horse from cold and wintry weather than it is from hot weather, humidity and blazing sun. Horses turned out in summer paddocks with no shelter to speak of are at risk of potentially fatal heatstroke, without doubt, or of freezing to death (especially the finer breeds) if they become really cold in winter. Horse clothing helps but must be very carefully monitored on horses or ponies out wearing it for long periods and two or three changes of clothing are needed so that dry, fairly clean rugs are always available. Good horse management demands that effective shelter from year-round weather is provided for horses who live out, and others should not be exposed to extremes of weather for sustained periods such as several hours.

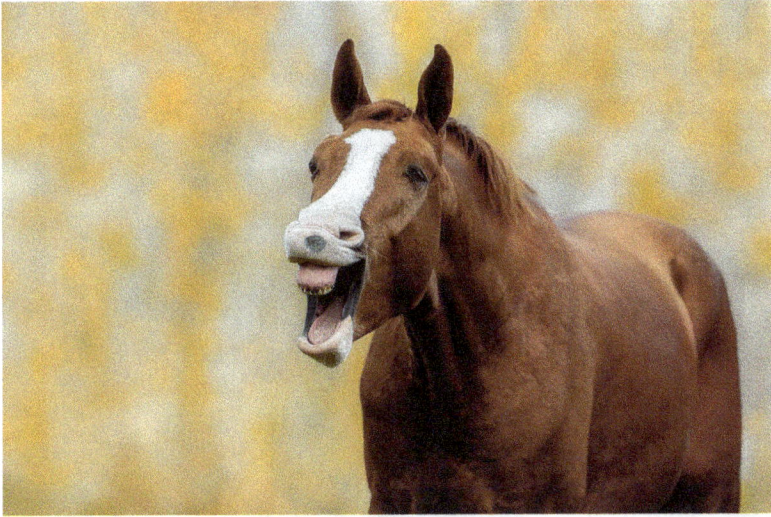

Figure 5.3 Like us and other animals, horses yawn when tired. Some say that they do it when stressed or short of oxygen, and it is safe to say that they do it when bored.
Source: (Shutterstock ID: 2191723513)

(It is often overlooked how damaging to a horse's feet and legs are squelching wet turnout areas, particularly when horses are on them for a long time. The ground becomes severely poached and damaged, grass growth is hampered, and horses can readily get mud fever which is very painful and can be difficult to treat, and not only on legs with white socks. Even regularly having to pass through a muddy gateway or stand in mud at a trough to access water can cause trouble or even put the horses off drinking at all.)

A healthy adult horse's normal temperature range is 99°F to 101°F or 37.2°C to 38.6°C. If the temperature varies above or below your horse's normal level by 1°F or ½°C, it is advisable to ring your veterinary surgeon for advice whether or not your horse is showing any signs of abnormal health and well-being.

Horses can survive very cold or hot temperatures in varied regions of the world, depending on their breed or type and, obviously, do so better with adequate shelter from both heat and cold, and carefully supervised clothing. This, however, is no reason to expect a clipped horse to live out in very hot or cold temperatures even wearing appropriate clothing. The summer coat is instrumental in helping to protect the skin from sunburn

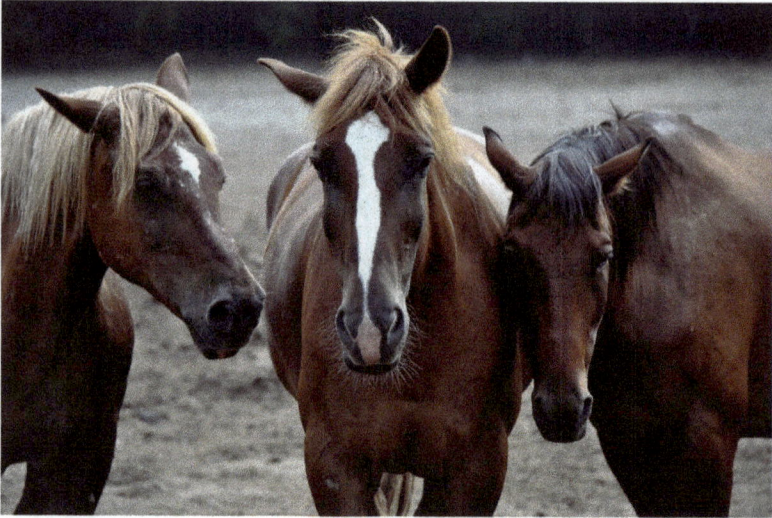

Figure 5.4 Three may be a crowd, but these horses are clearly happy and relaxed with their friends. They have calm expressions, their eyes are soft, ears relaxed held loosely to the sides or a little backwards and their nostrils relaxed. If they were alarmed or excited, this would show on their faces with wide-open eyes, ears firmly pricked towards whatever is catching their attention and their nostrils widely flared, trying to catch any scent that would help them identify the cause.
Source: (Shutterstock ID: 459413431)

and, of course, the winter one from cold, wind and wet conditions. Feral horses are obviously more able to acclimatise against weather conditions than domestic ones accustomed, even part-time, to the shelter of a stable or a good, well-sited field shelter-shed.

Signs of a horse feeling cold are shivering, looking hunched up, the coat 'staring' or standing away from the body (also a sign of illness), cold extremities, seeking shelter most of the time, standing by the paddock gate wanting to come in or even calling to be let in. A very cold horse's body temperature may well drop.

Signs of a horse feeling too hot are seeking shade, looking lethargic, being unsteady on his legs or actually staggering, lying flat out for extended periods (possibly actual heatstroke when the horse may become unconscious) and being hard to rouse. An over-heated horse's temperature will probably rise.

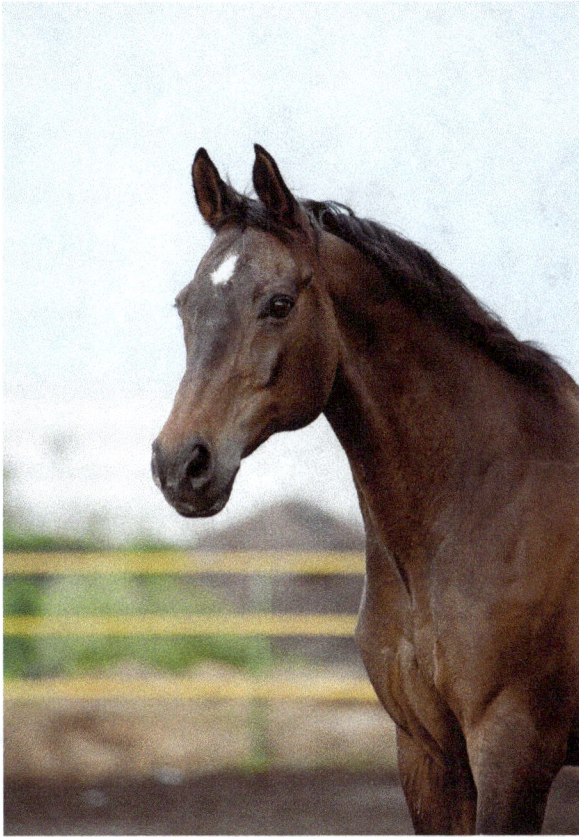

Figure 5.5 This horse is standing up still and alert, but not alarmed, at something ahead out of the picture. If he decides that it is not a threat his stance will become more relaxed, but if he decides otherwise his next step will be to run away from it if he possibly can.
Source: (Shutterstock ID: 107321642)

Heat is regulated to some extent by the coat trapping air next to the skin if a horse feels cold, and with a flat coat when he is comfortable or hot: he may well sweat if hot. Horses' bodies generate heat by means of their digestion of food within the intestines. Adequate food intake is, therefore, necessary to enable this. Hay is better for creating heat than concentrates, so horses out in cold weather should have full-time supplies of excellent quality hay provided, ideally in sheltered areas to protect the hay and allow horses to feel more comfortable while eating. Their diet can be topped up, if necessary, by feeding extra concentrates.

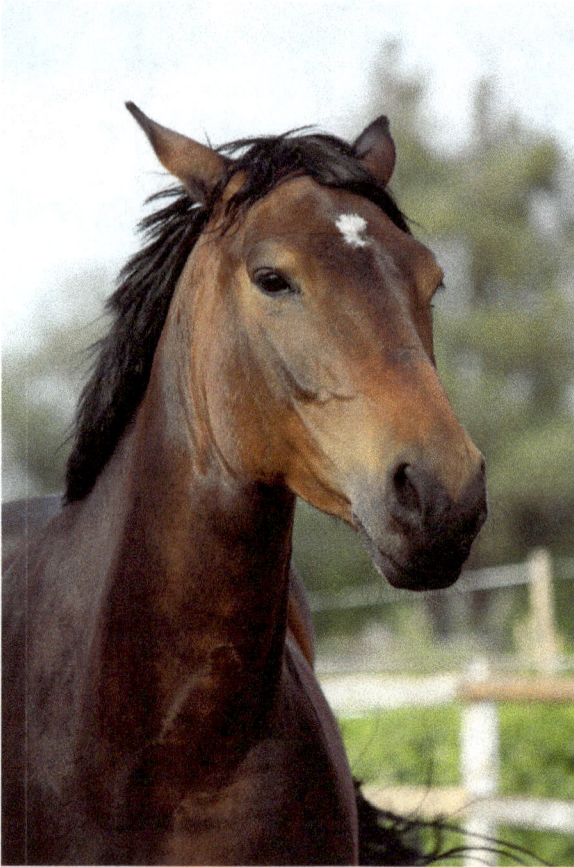

Figure 5.6 There is something behind this horse that is attracting his attention, but he is not worried by it, as shown by his ears pointed back to listen for information. He is not so bothered as to turn his head to look at whatever it is, his eyes are half closed and he remains quite calm.
Source: (Shutterstock ID: 78276211)

Vasodilation or expansion of the blood vessels is one means of allowing more heat, carried by the blood, to be lost through the skin. Conversely, constriction or narrowing of the vessels keeps the blood deeper within the body in cold conditions.

As well as heat and cold, horses can suffer from humidity. Although we, too, can feel this, I think we often under-estimate how, for instance, horses in poorly ventilated stables can suffer from it. I certainly usually get a splitting headache in hot, humid weather and who is to say horses don't? For horses, ideal humidity percentages are between 30 and

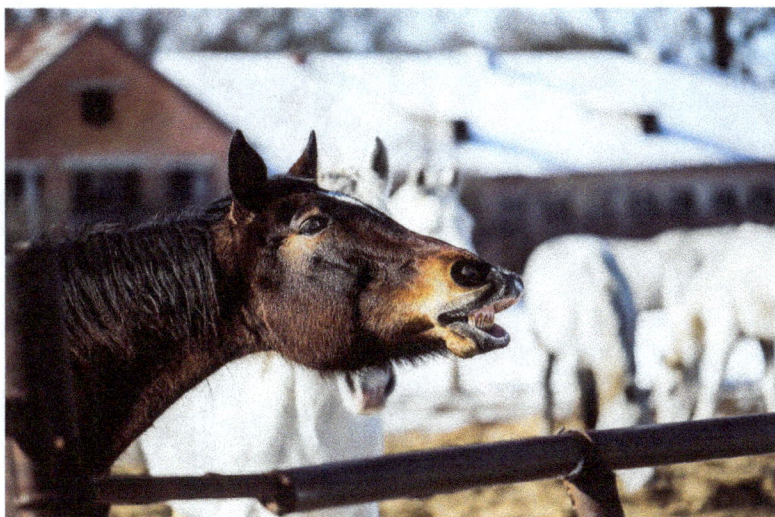

Figure 5.7 This is the *flehmen* response, which means 'to bare the front teeth'. Novice equestrians often think their horse is about to bite them! Flehmen is not a sign of anger and is not yawning. It is a specific action to identify smells for information and identification. The horse will breathe in air and, if it holds an unfamiliar or peculiar scent, will curl his upper lip up and back to help keep the air in the nostrils until his scent glands have familiarised him with it, or given him time to decide what it is. So it is basically a survival tactic. Horses might perform it when presented with unfamiliar food or bedding, or an unfamiliar object, person or horse, for instance. Stallions perform it to check whether or not a mare is in season. In this photograph, the horse has his eye on something or someone to his side and is trying to identify it.

Source: (Shutterstock ID: 2268062865)

50 per cent. As well as creating good ventilation in stables, it is an excellent plan to safely fit electric fans to help keep the horses cool. They can really appreciate this.

5.16 STEREOTYPICAL BEHAVIOURS

The distressing, repetitive actions we used to call 'stable vices' (as though the horse were at fault in performing them) are now looked on very differently. They are correctly called stereotypical behaviours and are a horse's psychological reaction to an unsuitable lifestyle for him or her as an individual. Contrary to the old belief, they are not 'catching' but very individual reactions to sustained distress.

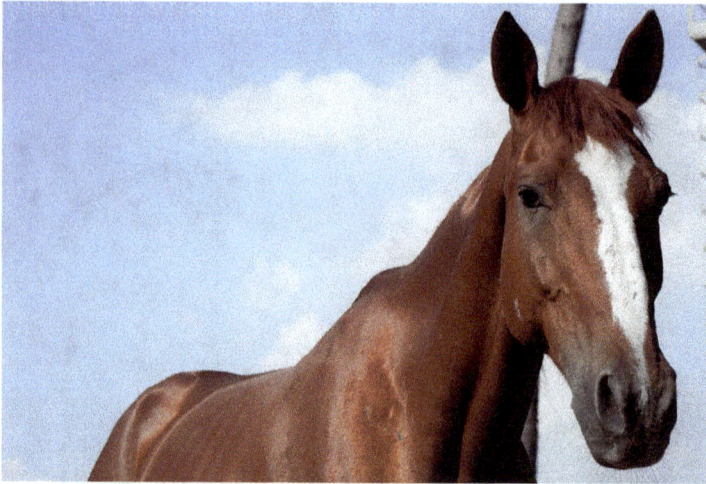

Figure 5.8 This horse is not happy at being alone. His ears are indicating his slight interest in the camera or photographer, but he is looking unhappy, dull and feeling 'down' because he is alone.
Source: (Shutterstock ID: 85225978)

It is almost always stabled horses who develop stereotypies rather than those living out, although the latter can develop swaying from side to side on their front hooves, often standing at the gate, as they yearn to be brought in. Horses who are already affected fairly strongly by stereotypies can certainly still perform them when turned out on tasty grazing with friends, although usually to a lesser extent.

Most of us will be familiar with one or more of these behaviours. They can be performed regularly or maybe occasionally when a horse is distressed or impatient about something, such as a neighbour having been taken out or being made to wait at feeding time, even the sight of the vet in the yard.

There is *crib-biting* in which the horse bites anything he can comfortably get his teeth on, such as the ledge formed by the tops of kicking boards or the top of his stable door. As he does this he may suck in air and make a honking or grunting noise. An extension of crib-biting is *wind-sucking* in which a horse performs the same action, possibly also with the noise, but does not need to bite on anything to help him. Wind-suckers often wave their heads up and down when performing this action. *Box walking* involves the horse walking round and round his box, often looking 'out of it' or not fully aware of his surroundings during the process. Another stereotypy is *weaving* in which the horse stands and sways from front hoof

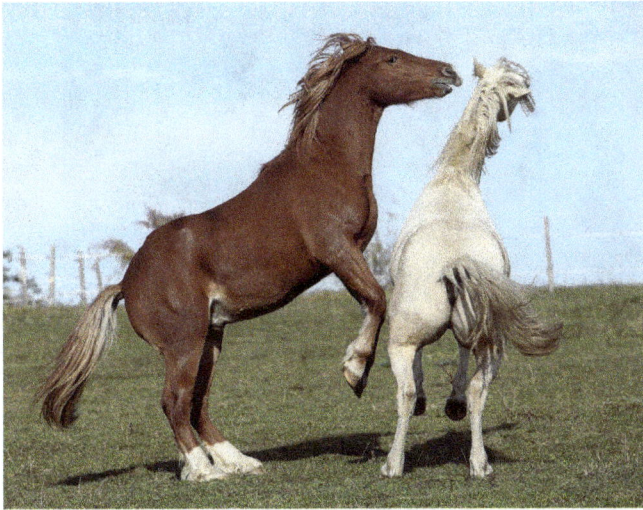

Figure 5.9 These two horses do not look as though they are having a fight (an actual fight between horses can be really frightening to witness). Horse play, though, can be rough. Mild high jinks like this are common and a usual part of equine communication. The horse on the left is striking out at the one on the right but does not look as though he means to hurt him. The horse on the right is inclining backwards to put himself safely out of reach of his companion's foreleg strike and raising his head out of reach of the hoof – and may well get his own back soon.
Source: (Shutterstock ID: 266998931)

to front hoof repeatedly, often looking over his stable door but sometimes inside his stable. These are the three main ones. Another is the horse swaying or throwing his head around repeatedly either over his stable door or inside the stable. There is also tongue-lolling and door kicking. Some people regard chewing clothing as a stereotypy, but others, myself included, feel it is just that the horse feels uncomfortable in his rug.

The general feeling is that stereotypical behaviours are impossible to cure. They can be lessened by making an affected horse as content as possible by making sure he has some food, such as hay, always available; his clothing is comfortable; he is stabled next to friendly horses, ideally his best friend/s; that the horses can touch each other in stables if at all possible and so on. It also helps to keep the horse interested in life, with an entertaining or pacifying view from his stable, friends with him or very close, plenty of enjoyable variety in his life, turnout, relaxed hacking and so on.

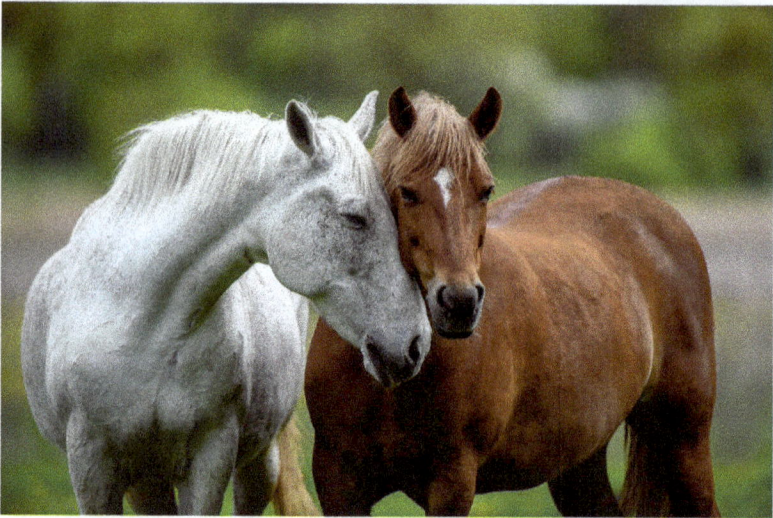

Figure 5.10 Two horses, grey on the left and chestnut on the right, heads together, eyes closed, showing great affection.
Source: (Shutterstock ID: 1993813604)

The old way of preventing horses performing their 'vices' in one way or another is now known to actually make them even more miserable because the various stereotypies they perform help them to bear the problems they perceive in their lives. When I was a child, any friend or classmate who, for instance, bit their nails, had their fingertips dipped in some foul-tasting liquid to stop them, which obviously made them more unhappy and only resulted in their developing some other action to replace it. Today, this is rightly condemned and behavioural counselling, I understand, is given to help the child. Treating horses in more understanding, modern ways, as discussed, is the way to deal with stereotypies, even though it may not be possible to entirely prevent them happening.

I know from my own experience that giving a horse a happier life and having him or her looked after and ridden by people whom he senses really care about his welfare and well-being goes a very long way to greatly reducing these behaviours, which may only then occur at occasional times like feeding times. Incidentally, it is best to feed affected horses first to relieve them, rather than keep to the old idea of making them wait as a punishment, an unkind and counter-productive attitude which only makes them worse.

The importance of the topics in, formerly, The Five Freedoms, now updated and entitled The Five Domains of Animal Welfare, cannot be over-estimated. For many millennia, humans have regarded animal life as of little importance and even regarded the animals themselves as insentient, unintelligent beings put on earth for the use of humans.

Of course, nothing could be further from the truth, although, and amazingly, it is only in recent decades that animals' ability to feel pain has been fully acknowledged. A similar situation exists with animal intelligence. It is only in very recent human generations that their undoubted intelligence has been acknowledged as being both different from and similar to our own, depending on their species. Many people in the world, strangely, do not think of humans as animals, yet clearly we are. We diverged from our ape ancestors millions of years ago yet we only have to look into the eyes of a chimpanzee or a bonobo, our closest ancestors, to see the close relationship.

Most horse enthusiasts know that the earliest equine ancestors were multi-toed, woodland-living mammals whose chance genetic mutations happened to fit them for a lifestyle on the newly developing plains. Their evolution into the horses we know today and the later evolution of modern humans were turning points in the very history of the Earth itself, for without Man's use of the family *equidae* the modern world and its history would have been very different.

As sentient beings, both horses and humans have a lot in common but with some remarkable differences. I hope very much that this book may have explained the value and importance of applying the organisation and clarity of The Five Domains of Animal Welfare to horses and ponies. Their care and management can be complicated and, if we get them wrong, they could die – at our hands. Although there are respected equestrian societies and organisations in most countries of the world, the problem is that they are run by humans – humans who very often have differing opinions as to what is right and wrong for the equines in their care.

The Five Domains set out a clear, rational, simple and reliable set of guidelines on looking after animals, and this book has both concentrated and expanded them into specifically equine requirements. When first-time owners buy a horse they frequently take advice from horse-owning friends or acquaintances, their local riding schools where they still exist or, increasingly, social media with all its risks and confusions. I hope very much that the contents of this book will act as a clear guide to the particular topics that are the most important in equine care and management.

There will be times when you need more help or advice concerning your horses or ponies and, here, I sincerely suggest that you do not confuse yourself by becoming sucked in to the countless and often mind-boggling opinions expressed on social media. Apart from the obvious necessity of a superb equine veterinary surgeon, the horse world now has a dazzling array of qualified, specialist equine practitioners in just about every field you could think of. As well as vets and farriers, we have physiotherapists, masseurs, shiatsu practitioners, behavioural consultants and tack fitters. The best feed companies have free telephone advice services from qualified equine nutritionists who can be most helpful. Of course, we also have riding teachers and coaches qualified to various levels, although I should prefer to see a clear move in their training towards Equitation Science

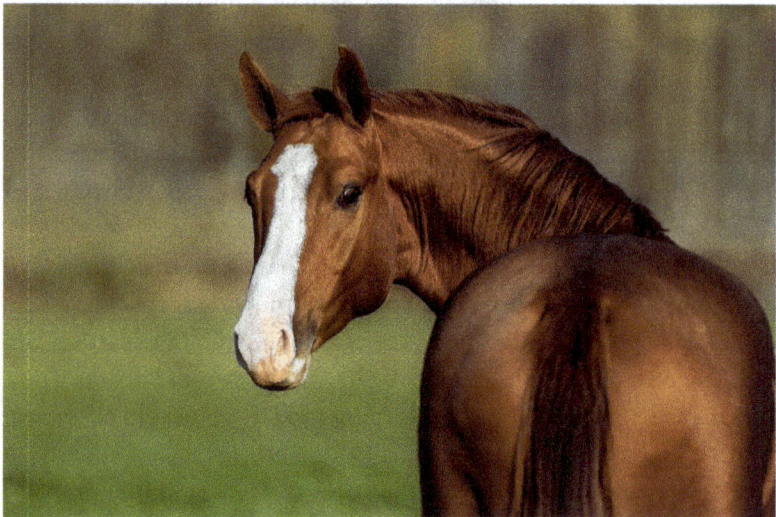

Figure A.1 'Bye!'

principles and, as ever, those of true classical riding (see my book *Fine Riding* published by CRC Press/Taylor & Francis).

Whatever you wish to do with your horse or pony, I wish you both much pleasure together, plus that magical element of a large slice of good luck when you need it most.

Susan McBane

Index

Note: Page numbers in *italics* indicate a figure on the corresponding page.

For Product Safety Concerns and Information please contact our EU
representative GPSR@taylorandfrancis.com
Taylor & Francis Verlag GmbH, Kaufingerstraße 24, 80331 München, Germany

www.ingramcontent.com/pod-product-compliance
Lightning Source LLC
Chambersburg PA
CBHW050520280326
41932CB00014B/2393